Praise for The Powerful She

"My name is Maurice Benard.
The Powerful She is all about state of mind.
You have to believe in yourself.
And this book is all about empowering yourself.
Don't forget, you women are amazing."

~ Maurice Benard
Three-time Emmy Award winner All My Children

THE POWERFUL
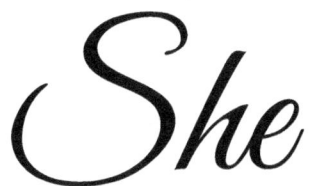

Stories of 18 Women with
LOVE GRACE COURAGE

Curated By

Liza Boubari

Copyright © 2025 Liza Boubari

Visit the author's website at www.thepowerfulshe.com

THE POWERFUL SHE

All rights reserved. No part of this publication may be reproduced, distributed, or transmitted in any form or by any means, including photocopying, recording, or other electronic or mechanical methods, without the prior written permission of the publisher, except in the case of brief quotations embodied in critical reviews and certain other noncommercial uses permitted by United States of America copyright law and fair use. For permission requests, write to the publisher, "Attention: Permissions Coordinator," at info@healwithin.com.

ISBN 978-1-7333126-6-0 (print)

ISBN 978-1-7333126-5-3 (epub)

Library of Congress Control Number: 2024926630

Second Edition

Published by HealWithin, Inc.
330 Arden Ave Suite 130
Glendale CA 91203
www.healwithin.com

Dedication

You know the routine: you open a book, turn to the dedication, and find it devoted to someone else.

Not this time.

This book is dedicated to you—the women in this book and our collective lineage: the mothers, daughters, sisters, and ancestors whose choices, challenges, and triumphs paved the way for us to be here today.

Though we may never meet in person, we've already connected through these words, stories, and chapters. Each story weaves a thread of our shared experience—some may mirror your own journey, others may feel like distant echoes. Yet all of them, including yours, hold power. Your story matters. Your voice deserves to be written, heard and celebrated.

Let this book be a reminder: not only do I Matter and She Matters, but You Matter—in all your complexity, strength, and beauty.

For you, for her, for all of us.

Table of Contents

FORWARD 3

INTRODUCTION 8

HEALWITHIN 12

    Evoke – Embrace – Evolve
    LIZA BOUBARI

UNLEASHING THE POWER WITHIN 31

    A Journey of Love, Resilience, and Extraordinary Events
    LINDA CAIN

MILLIONS & MINEFIELDS 43

    Trapped by Expectation
    TIFFANY CUI

THE UNVEILING 54

    CARL-A DIRAN

RESILIENCE UNLEASHED 65

    A Woman's Rise to Empowerment
    LADY JEN DU PLESSIS

MY JOURNEY INTO FUTURES 76

    MANOUSHAG (MAY) EMIRZIAN

A LIFE FULL OF CHANCES, CHOICES, AND CHANGES 86

    ARMINA GHARPETIAN

THE RESILIENCE OF LOVE 93

    JENNIFER L. HORSPOOL

STITCHED IN FATE 107

ZARIK KAZANCHIAN

THE POWER OF LOVE 117

The #FreeBritney Movement and Me
LISA MACCARLEY

WANDERING WIND 130

SANAZ MANOUCHEHRIAN

AGAINST ALL ODDS 142

The Journey of Turning My Mess into My Message
ALINA MARTIN

DISCOVERING THE POWERFUL SHE IN ME 154

NANCY MATTHEWS

SINGLE FLOWER IN A CONCRETE STREET 165

GIA RAZANDO

OVERCOMING OBSTACLES AND PEAKS 179

NATALIE REGG

BREAKING BARRIERS, INSPIRING CHANGE 192

BAYDSAR THOMASIAN

GUIDED BY FAITH 207

A Journey of Resilience, Compassion, and Inspiration
IRMA VILLEGAS

TO ARMENIA, WITH LOVE 219

LIANA TOMEKYAN

* * *

Forward

By **Dr. Ani Kalayjian**
Bestselling author and CEO of MeaningfulWorld

The Powerful She is like a warm sun breaking through the clouds, illuminating a path of resilience, courage, and transformation. With heartfelt dedication, Liza Boubari has curated a profound collection of stories that guide us to embrace our inner power and strength and the lessons learned from life's challenges.

I have known Liza for years, and although our connection began virtually, our shared passion for healing and empowerment has brought us closer. Liza is not only a clinical hypnotherapist and founder of HealWithin but also a compassionate, heart-centered leader who uplifts others with grace and perseverance. Her vision for The Powerful She is selfless and bold, celebrating unsung heroines and their transformative journeys.

The stories within this book reflect universal struggles and triumphs, weaving together pain and healing, fear and courage, despair, and hope. Each chapter aligns beautifully with the 7-step Integrative Healing Model that has been at the core of my work in trauma recovery and post-traumatic growth:

1. Identifying and understanding negative emotions (emotional intelligence).
2. Releasing and achieving catharsis.
3. Feeling validated and receiving empathy to foster closure.
4. Shifting toward meaning-making and learning positive lessons.
5. Sharing tools and resources for healing and forgiveness.
6. Connecting with Mother Earth for ecological intelligence.

7. Engaging in physical and spiritual practices for balance and renewal.

Through these steps, the authors reveal how they've turned trauma into wisdom, suffering into service, and challenges into opportunities for growth. Each story is a sunrise waiting to be witnessed, offering courage, grace, and tools for transformation.

- Alina's story teaches us the power of inclusion and resilience in transforming physical challenges into poetry and purpose.
- Armina's journey from political violence to flourishing as a dentist and mentor highlights the strength found in faith and family.
- Baydsar's experience of overcoming cancer and advocating for her community exemplifies post-traumatic growth through service.
- Carla's story reveals how healing from generational and childhood trauma leads to self-respect and inner peace.
- Gia's breakthrough from abuse to healing through love and systemic constellation shows the power of releasing pain.
- Irma's faith-driven path through immigration, bullying, and family struggles inspires us to embrace hope and service.
- Jen's courage to confront her past and find her voice reminds us that leadership begins within.
- Jennifer's journey of overcoming distrust and embracing self-love offers tools for generational healing.
- Liana's transformation through cancer and creating Satik's Home in Armenia exemplifies resilience and giving back.
- Linda's life of bringing people together and adopting six children embodies love, leadership, and connection.
- Lisa's advocacy in the #FreeBritney movement shows how passion and purpose can spark global change.
- Liza's personal story of healing and empowering others reflects her profound courage and compassion.

- Manoushag's trading journey highlights the importance of aligning beliefs with goals and embracing persistence.
- Nancy's reframing of trading into a positive venture shows the power of trust and self-belief.
- Natalie's outdoor adventures reveal how breaking stereotypes empowers women and builds confidence.
- Sanaz's resilience through political, individual, and generational traumas reminds us of the strength of helping others.
- Tiffany's leadership path exemplifies how coaching others to purpose begins with embracing your growth.
- Zarik's determination to overcome visual challenges inspires us to believe in prayer, grace, and self-trust.

These remarkable women remind us of Rumi's words: "Never lose hope, my heart; miracles dwell in the invisible." Together, they transform trauma into wisdom, despair into hope, and struggles into triumphs.

May this book inspire you to explore your own path of transformation and embrace the courage to heal, love, and live with purpose. As we say at MeaningfulWorld, "Shared sorrow is half sorrow, while shared joy is double joy!"

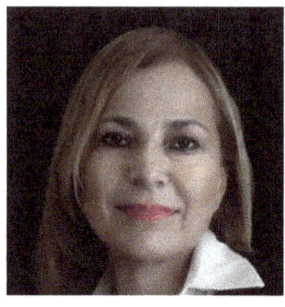 **Dr. Ani Kalayjian**
Board Certified Expert in Traumatic Stress
Fellow of the New York Academy of Medicine
Fellow of the American Psychological Association
Ambassador, Psi Chi, Honor Society in Psychology
Adj. Professor of Psychology, Teachers College, Columbia University
President, Association for Trauma Outreach & Prevention
United Nations Representative
Integrative Healer, http://drkalayjian.com
Founder and President, http://meaningfulworld.com/

Author of 6 books, including *7 Steps for Healing Our Body, Mind, Spirit, and Mother Earth*; *Forgiveness & Reconciliation*, *Mass Trauma & Emotional Healing around the World (2 Volumes)*; *A Journey for Empowerment, Healing & Transformation*.

Introduction
The Powerful She

Welcome to *The Powerful She*, a captivating anthology that weaves together women's narratives on a profound journey of self-discovery and empowerment, each story a testament to resilience and triumph over adversity.

In conceiving this collaboration, my vision was to illuminate the stories of remarkable women—individuals whose successes and talents often lay obscured beneath layers of self-doubt, limiting beliefs, and societal expectations, resonating with you and me.

Every woman, including yourself, possesses a unique story—a compelling narrative enriched by the formidable challenges faced and conquered against all odds. This collection isn't just about the stories; it's about what lies beneath them—the innate ability we share to build connections, foster collaboration, invite love into our hearts, and summon the grace and courage needed to heal from within.

The Powerful She represents a diverse spectrum of talents and gifts historically underestimated or overlooked due to societal norms and gender stereotypes. I firmly believe that "to give in is my weakness—to give up is my choice."

Within these pages, you'll unravel tales of trials confronted, obstacles surmounted, and unwavering determination that fuels the journeys of these inspiring women. Through laughter, tears, and moments of sheer triumph, you'll witness the beauty of the human spirit rising above adversity as each woman taps into her feminine energy and inner strength to Show Up, Stand Up, and Speak Up.

I hope that, within the chapters, you'll find something that resonates with you—a story that sparks inspiration, prompts a new choice, or instigates a shift within because you matter.

The Powerful She is more than a collection of stories; it's a celebration of the universal power women possess to create change, find purpose, and touch the lives of those around them. As you embark on this journey through the narratives, you'll be captivated by the authenticity, vulnerability, and strength that resonates within the shared experiences of sisterhood.

Love, Grace, and Courage: The Triad of Empowerment

This anthology celebrates three core virtues that weave through the fabric of these women's lives: Love, Grace, and Courage.

Love: The Essence of Human Existence

Love empowers us to lead with our hearts, make decisions based on compassion, and embrace the essence of our humanity. Women have a unique ability to express and embody this emotion, forging deep connections, fostering empathy, and nurturing relationships.

Grace: The Elegance of Inner Peace

Grace emanates from within, embodying elegance, poise, and dignity. Women who embrace grace carry themselves with a sense of inner peace, navigating adversity with tact and diplomacy and fostering self-acceptance and self-love.

Courage: The Catalyst for Change

Courage propels women to break free from limitations, conquer fears, and embrace their full potential. It empowers them to face challenges head-on, step outside their comfort zones, and become catalysts for change.

Living with Love, Grace, and Courage requires inner strength, resilience, self-awareness, a commitment to personal growth, and a willingness to embrace vulnerability. Embodying these virtues, we acknowledge that the journey is not always easy, but the rewards far outweigh the challenges.

Maya Angelou aptly reminds us, *"Each time a woman stands up for herself, without knowing it possibly, without claiming it, she stands up for all women."*

Let *The Powerful She* be a beacon of inspiration, a testament to intelligent, courageous, and loving women who teach by being. Remember, "I Matter – You Matter – She Matters," and collectively, We Matter.

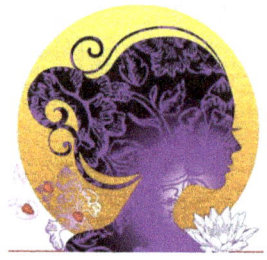

The Symbolism of the cover of The Powerful She
- The Sun – Yellow represents the life cycle and the center and core of our body.
- The Woman – beautiful just as she is, looking into the future (the left, which represents our feminine energy-receiving side).
- The Black – indicates all the complex challenges we endure and overcome.
- The Purple is associated with royalty, luxury, ambition, wealth, creativity, wisdom, dignity, devotion, peace, pride, and independence. It is associated with the third eye, which allows us to see the bigger picture and gain wisdom.
- The Lotus symbolizes purity, strength, resilience, and rebirth because lotuses rise from the mud without stains.
- The Pomegranate symbolizes fertility and abundance. It is a symbol of life. Each mature Pomegranate has 365 seeds, one for each day of the year.
- The Powerful She is a reminder of the hidden powers within us that ought to be revealed and shared with Love, grace, and courage.

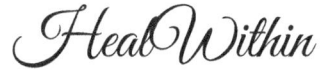

Heal Within
EVOKE – EMBRACE – EVOLVE
Liza Boubari

The Powerful She: A Glimpse into My Story

Once upon a time, nestled among the towering mountains of uptown Tehran, there lived a little girl with a radiant smile and a heart brimming with dreams. Her spirit was gregarious yet gentle, but beneath her sunny disposition lay a hidden reservoir of pain that she concealed even from herself.

That little girl was me.

From the outside, my childhood might have looked perfect. I had pretty dresses, a loving family, and a home filled with stories and laughter. But I also carried a scar—a small, blue line above my lip—that I believed made me look like the ugly duckling. My mom kept my hair short with bangs while other girls flaunted long, braided locks. Their beauty seemed effortless, while I constantly felt "not pretty enough." Isn't it remarkable how early those feelings creep into a young girl's heart?

What about you?

Can you think back to when you ever believed you weren't enough? Maybe it was because of how you looked, spoke, or how others treated you. How did that moment make you feel?

We, as women, are often taught to put on a brave face. To say, "I'm Ok or fine," when everything inside us feels as if coming apart or broken. But here's what I want you to know: You are not your scars, your fears, or your failures. You are so much more.

The Women Who Shaped Me

My family's story is a tapestry of survival, resilience, and transformation. My maternal grandparents survived the Armenian Genocide of 1915, carrying the weight of unimaginable trauma. My paternal grandparents, a mix of Turkish and born in Baku, carried their complexities. Together, these two worlds created a foundation that was rich, complicated, and beautiful.

Among the many powerful figures in my life, my grandmother Roza (Rosaline) stood out as a beacon of love and resilience. Born in 1907, Roza experienced the horrors of the Armenian Genocide firsthand. Despite witnessing unspeakable horrors, her courage and strength were evident in how she carried herself, with a quiet dignity that spoke volumes about her resilience. Every wrinkle on her hands and face told a story of survival and courage, and her eyes sparkled with a mixture of sorrow and hope.

While Roza's experiences had undoubtedly shaped her, they did not harden her heart. She remained innocent and pure. She possessed a childlike wonder and curiosity about the world, which I find in myself.

Grandma taught me that no matter what life takes from you, it cannot take your spirit—unless you let it. She found joy in the smallest things, like singing songs in multiple languages or playing the piano. Even at 59, she learned to drive and bought herself a blue Fiat, proving it's never too late to reclaim your independence.

My strength, innocence, and love are because of who she was. She taught me the importance of resilience in the face of adversity, the power of maintaining integrity despite life's hardships, and the transformative nature of love and being of service.

My loving mother, the youngest of four, grew up shouldering immense responsibility. Mom has a quality that exudes elegance, poise, and dignity. She possesses an innate elegance and poise that allows her to face adversity with resilience and maintain a sense of composure in the face of turmoil.

Mom, then Mary Sarkissian, was crowned Miss Airport in 1958. She was the first female flight attendant to fly with the Shah of Iran. Perhaps my love for flying started then! I also attribute my passion for reading, being graceful yet proper, love for fashion, caring, and compassion for the needs of others to my mother. Her decorum masked an inner warrior who faced life's challenges head-on.

Although critical at times, her gracefulness extends to her interactions with others, offering kindness, understanding, and empathy even under challenging circumstances.

These two women taught me that strength doesn't mean being unbreakable. It means being able to pick up the pieces, no matter how many times you've been shattered.

In the midst of darkness- find your inner light. Our eyes are not only to see but to project what we witness.
You Matter ~Liza

Evoke: The Body Keeps the Score

In my twenties, I began to experience recurring ovarian cysts, a physical manifestation of the unprocessed pain I carried within. After two surgeries, I found myself once again in a doctor's office, hearing the dreaded words: "You have another cyst."

At that moment, I heard nothing else – not a word of what he was saying – not the sounds outside – as if I was no longer in the same room. Everything else became a blur. I do not recall how I left the doctor's office; I only remember walking down the hallway and replaying what he had just told me.

Due to my history and how fast the cysts grew, he recommended scheduling surgery in less than a month. I remember the sordid faces staring at me in the elevator. Tears streamed down my face as I sat alone in the car afterward, consumed by memories of shame, loss, and inadequacy. I longed for a child, yet my body seemed to betray me at every turn. The harsh words of my ex-husband echoed in my mind: "You can't get pregnant because God doesn't think you're worthy of being a mother." Those words and others became chains, tightening around my throat and chest.

I cried my heart out – not because I had developed another cyst, or it could be cancerous, or that it was anything worse, but hear this: I was crying because I'd longed for and been wanting a baby for so long – the last thing I needed was yet another cyst growing in me. This would be the third time... they say three is a charm...but nothing seemed charming then.

But amidst the darkness, a quiet yet powerful voice arose within me. It whispered: Enough. No more. That moment of clarity changed everything. I realized I didn't need another surgery. What I needed was to truly heal—not just my body, but my spirit.

Now you can understand how ridiculous this was. Sitting in my car and having all these memories and thoughts, even emotions, coming up to the point that I felt my heart beating fast and new, then - here it goes, another anxiety attack is coming.

Have you ever felt like your body was trying to tell you something? Maybe through a persistent ache, a sickness, or even fatigue? Our bodies hold onto everything we suppress. Every tear we don't cry, every word we don't say, every hurt we try to ignore—it all finds a place in our bodies.

What is your body trying to tell you?

My Promise

We immigrated to the United States when I was 16. In middle school, I was one of 15 Armenians. In those early times, I was quite self-conscious and faced relentless bullying. Some teased me about my accent, how I dressed, how I walked—just because I was different. Desperate to fit in, I traded my European and proper dresses for jeans and T-shirts, stuck a comb in my back pocket, and I even carried cigarettes in my backpack. By age 14, I was already smoking cigarettes—this attempt to blend in spiraled into a story of its own.

There was a bridge near our middle school where the kids who smoked gathered at lunchtime. One day, I was walking there with my new friends Karl, Mark, Shannon, and Janet—they made me feel safe and like I belonged. This one day, Stephanie, the leader of the girls' gang, stood in my way. With a sneer, she dared me to smoke what she held in her hand if I wanted to pass. I was trembling inside, but I didn't let her see my fear. I took a puff, held back the cough, and exhaled as if it were just another cigarette. She smirked, nodded, and let me through.

After lunch, in my favorite art class with Ms. Jo Willoughby, I started giggling uncontrollably. What I didn't realize at the time was that what I smoked had just hit me. My giggles turned to laughter so intense that I nearly gagged. Ms. Willoughby, a kind and caring teacher with the most beautiful smile, asked me to step out of the classroom. Outside, she took my hands, looked me in the eyes, and said something that would stay with me forever:

"Liza, you are such a beautiful, intelligent, and talented girl. Did you smoke something during lunch? I shook my head as if yes. Next, she asked if I would tell her who gave it to me, and I shook my head no. Then she said this: Ok... I want you to know you don't need this to feel good. Promise me you'll never take or smoke anything like that again."

In that moment, I felt truly seen and cared for. With tears in my eyes, I squeezed her hand and said, "Yes, I promise." It took me years to realize how specific memories and experiences shape the trajectory of our lives. That promise became a turning point in my life. Years later, I realized how such moments—rooted in raw emotion—can imprint on the subconscious and shape who we become. That promise was kept to this day.

Age 5-6.

I have a black-and-white picture of myself, which is about five or six years old. In it, I'm wearing a cowboy hat, a holster strapped to my waist, and toy guns at my side. I look ready—confident, fierce as if I could take on the world. But the truth behind that picture is something I've never spoken about. I wanted to hurt those who hurt me.

When I was about five or six, a distant family member abused me. It didn't happen just once—it happened again and again. And every time, I was warned: "Don't tell anyone. If you do, they won't believe you, and the punishment will be worse." So, I stayed silent.

I carried the fear with me like a weight, heavy and constant. I buried it deep inside because I was too afraid to speak out, too scared of what "worse" could mean. That silence became a part of me. It seeped into everything I did, shaping the way I saw myself and the way I moved through the world.

Age 7. In class, I didn't understand the subject, so I whispered a question to my friend. Before I could finish, the teacher's sharp voice cut through the room, calling my name.

"Stand up!" she demanded, her eyes cold and unyielding. My heart pounded as she asked me to recite what she had just explained. My mind was blank. I couldn't answer.

Frustrated, she ordered, "Go to the back of the room! Stand in the corner—one leg up." The faint giggles of my classmates followed as I stumbled to the corner. Staring at the cracks in the paint, I tried to focus to stop the tears from falling. My raised leg began to ache, and I finally lowered it for balance.

Her voice boomed. "Put your leg back up!" My tears spilled over as I begged, "Please, I need to go to the bathroom." She didn't believe me, accusing me of lying. And then it happened—the warmth spread down my legs.

The humiliation was complete. Without a word, she grabbed my arm and dragged me out of the classroom. Tears streamed down my face the entire time.

Age 11. Sitting at my desk, working on a math problem, my tutor explained multiplication. At first, everything seemed normal. Then his hand moved to my leg.

It started gently, almost imperceptible, but became deliberate and slow. My stomach churned, and I tried to shift away. His hand followed.

He leaned closer, smiling. "Stay still and be a good girl. Don't you want to pass this class?"

I froze. All I could think was, I do. I want to pass. I stayed still—not because I wanted to, but because I didn't know how to make it stop.

At that moment, I hated him. I hated math. And I hated myself for not knowing how to fight back.

These moments lingered like shadows I couldn't escape. The fear, the shame, the helplessness—they became part of who I was.

For years, I carried them silently, pretending they didn't matter. But they did.

Years later, talking with friends about school, we realized he had failed some of us deliberately, forcing summer tutoring with the same predatory tactics. None of us ever told our parents.

If you've ever felt trapped like this, carrying pain too heavy to share, know this: You are not alone.

Stop carrying it silently. You are more than what happened to you. You are stronger than fear, shame, or silence. You Matter.

The Lesson

Life has taught me those specific moments—both painful and profound—can shape the trajectory of our lives. A simple promise, made in a moment of vulnerability, can plant the seeds for transformation. For me, that transformation began with the courage to say No more.

This is the message I carry forward: We all have the power to honor the promises we make to ourselves and to choose a path of strength, clarity, and self-respect.

Embrace: Transforming Pain into Power

Healing is rarely straightforward. It can be messy and requires facing truths we've spent years avoiding. My journey began when I learned to listen—not just to my thoughts, but to my body.

For so long, I carried pain without questioning it. It simply was. But during a pivotal hypnotherapy session, my practitioner suggested something unexpected: "Talk to your pain. Ask it what it needs." Skeptical but desperate, I closed my eyes and tried.

To my surprise, my pain answered.

It wasn't there to harm me but to protect me. It wasn't the enemy—it was a messenger carrying years of unspoken fears, denied anger, and buried shame.

At that moment, I realized that the body doesn't lie. It remembers everything—heartbreaks, betrayals, and the emotions we avoid. And when it can't bear the weight anymore, it whispers through discomfort and pain. The question is, are we willing to listen?

That day, I chose to listen. For the first time, I didn't fight against my body. I didn't silence it or push it away. Instead, I let it guide me, unraveling the tightly wound threads of my emotions. With every tear that fell, with every memory that surfaced, I began to understand that healing wasn't about fixing myself. It was about embracing myself—pain and all.

It wasn't an overnight transformation, but it was a beginning. By listening to the wisdom within, I found the strength to move forward.

The 3E Event

In this spirit, I founded The 3E Events, a transformative day of healing, connection, and empowerment. For nine years, I brought women together to interact with like-minded souls, experience healing exercises, and celebrate life through music and dance. These events were filled with the energy of shared stories and the inspiration of powerful speakers who delivered impactful messages of growth, courage, and self-love. Together, we created a space where women could reconnect with their inner strength and realize they were not alone on their journey.

And that is why I have now dedicated myself to creating intimate retreats to help others heal within. These retreats are to be a space to reconnect—mind, body, spirit, and nature—and to begin the transformative journey of self-discovery and self-love.

For those seeking something smaller but equally profound, I offer workshops I call 'Listen to Your Body Talk.' In these workshops, we learn breathwork and self-hypnosis, explore the signals our bodies give us, uncover the emotions hidden beneath the surface, and learn how to embrace our inner wisdom.

Because healing isn't just about moving past pain, it's about listening, honoring, and connecting with the very core of who we are.

And so, I invite you to listen to your body, to its whispers and its wisdom. You might be surprised at what it has to say. Contact me to take part in our workshops or retreats.

Embracing Strength

My father often said in Farsi, "Baraye kee, baraye chee?"— which translates to "For whom, and for what?"

As a child, I heard it as a challenge, dismissing my desires and questioning their worth. But as I've grown, I now see it differently. It was never meant to diminish anything, especially me. It was a call—a question of purpose, of intention. What truly matters? And why?

One day, lost in the flood of memories, something shifted inside me. I remembered his words. It wasn't a roar—it was a whisper. But it was unshakable.

That's it! I now know my why. I do it to share my experience to make a difference."

The voice was mine, powerful and resolute, and it refused to be ignored. At that moment, I remembered the promise I made to Ms. Willoughby all those years ago. Her words had saved me and ignited something in me. If I could promise her, why couldn't I promise myself? And so I did.

I turned it to: "Baraye man – Baraye hame." —which translates to: "For me and them all." That promise became my strength, my anchor. To this day, I am reminded of one unassailable truth: I deserved better. I Matter. You Matter. We Matter

Evolve: A New Chapter

As Women, We Must Stop Hiding. As women, we're not here to merely exist—we're here to express boldly and authentically. Yet, too often, we hide behind smiles, burying our pain and fears, afraid of judgment or vulnerability.

But here's the truth: You are better than that.

You are a child of God, with a magic and power uniquely yours. You were created to shine, not to shrink or silence your voice. Being authentic means saying, "This is who I am, scars and all."

Yes, vulnerability is scary—but it's also your greatest strength. When you share your truth, you not only heal yourself but create space for others to heal, too. In every challenge, there's a gift. In every struggle, an opportunity.

What would it feel like to stop pretending and let the world see the real you—the beautiful, imperfect, powerful you?

Evoke, Embrace, Evolve: The 3E Woman

To the woman reading this: I see you. I see your pain, your struggles, your doubts. And I want you to know this—you are not alone. Whatever you've been through, whatever you're carrying, it doesn't have to define you. It can shape you, but it doesn't have to control you.

Our experiences, no matter how painful, don't have to define us as trauma forever. They can become the foundation for growth, resilience, and transformation when we heal from the inside out. That's exactly the beauty of HealWithin: guiding individuals to not just cope with the past but to release it, embrace their present, and evolve into their fullest potential.

You are a 3E Woman. You matter. Your story matters. The pain you've endured, the battles you've fought, and the scars you carry—they are all part of your journey. But they are not your destination.

Today Is Your Beginning - To live victoriously, you must confront the stories that hold you back. Face your challenges and step into your truth. It's time to

Evoke your passion: Speak your truth. Your dreams and feelings matter.

Embrace your femininity: Celebrate the strength and wisdom within you.

Evolve spiritually: Become who you've always been—a woman of power and grace.

Healing begins within. It's not about erasing the past but transforming it into a foundation for growth. With grace, courage, and self-love, you can choose today to be the day you let go of what no longer serves you. You can choose to embrace your inner power and create a life filled with purpose and joy.

Remember: When you are ready to evoke what was, embrace what is, and evolve into what can be, you'll discover the truth—you are the Powerful She.

With Gratitude,

Liza

Liza Boubari

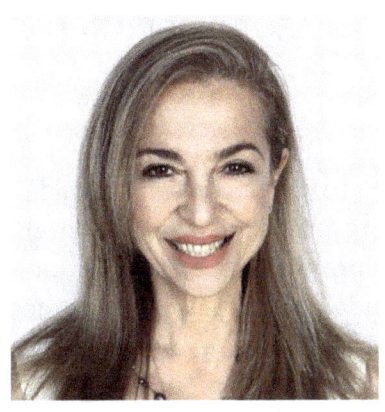

Liza Boubari is a celebrated author, dynamic motivational speaker, and women's wellness expert with over 24 years of experience empowering individuals to heal within. Her transformative journey began with her powerful healing experience through hypnotherapy, which inspired her to leave a career in the corporate world and dedicate her life to helping others. In 1999, Liza founded HealWithin, Inc., a sanctuary for personal growth and emotional well-being.

As the author of numerous books, including Heal-Thy Mind-Body and Stand Up to Slim Down, Stomp on Smoking, and creator of over a dozen hypnosis audios, Liza's work is a testament to her dedication to guiding others toward positive transformation. Her expertise spans mindfulness, emotional resilience, and self-empowerment, and her passion lies in giving women a voice and helping them share their stories.

Liza is a radio personality and hosts *Real-Talk with Liza* on AM870, where she blends heartfelt conversations with actionable guidance to inspire women to move forward confidently. Her mission is simple yet profound: to empower women to recognize their inner power, share their unique voices, and create lives of meaning and fulfillment.

Ready to embark on your journey of transformation? Connect with Liza for immersive healing retreats, apply to share your story on *Real-Talk with Liza*, or work with her one-on-one to reclaim your power and purpose. Your healing chapter starts here.

Website: https://www.HealWithin.com
Facebook: https://www.facebook.com/boubari
Instagram: https://www.instagram.com/lizaboubari/
LinkedIn: https://www.linkedin.com/in/healwithin/

Unleashing the Power Within
A JOURNEY OF LOVE, RESILIENCE, AND EXTRAORDINARY EVENTS
Linda Cain

Introduction

In "The Powerful She," I invite you to dive into my life's wild rollercoaster! Explore the captivating journey of a woman (me) whose passion for events has transformed lives, businesses, and entire communities. My name is Linda Cain, and I am a seasoned event planner, the founder and CEO of Blu Diamond Event Management, friend, confidant, and your best cheerleader! Throughout my professional career spanning over two decades, I have specialized in entrepreneurship, creating extraordinary experiences for clients worldwide. I have produced or participated in over 1200 events of all kinds. But there's more to me than name tags, itineraries, and locations. I'm also a wife, mom, friend, and entrepreneur. A woman who has seen it all and lived to plan another party. This chapter follows my journey far beyond business; it encompasses love, family, compassion, and resilience that have shaped who I am today.

Youth, Dreams, and the Road to Serving Others

From the outset, I knew I was destined for a career in events. Even during high school, as a cheerleader who helped organize competitions and rallies, I always loved seeing people come together. I was not the kind of person who sat at home. I loved being out and about with others, and thanks to many hustles, some lucky breaks, and a clipboard in my hand, things fell into place. By the time I graduated high school, I had worked as a highly paid babysitter (even taking CPR classes and officially babysitting classes), worked with a catering company supporting weddings and parties, and worked in a restaurant and for a pharmacy.

Being part of events at an early age also allowed me to get to know and experience different cultures and people from all walks of life. I loved this!

My mom used to call me a "chum" magnet, and my friends used to call me an "old soul." At an early age, I seemed to have the knack to step into different situations and defuse, calm, support, and see the bigger picture.

I was the kind of kid whom others came to talk about their friends and why they were not included on party invitations, or why the "boy" didn't like them, or how to get a "girl" to like them. My loyalties were fierce, and I could hold confidence. My teachers and other adults also would involve me in conversations that, looking back, were on a higher level.

This led me to be the kind of friend that made others feel safe. I kept the calmness of the pep squad during competitions. I was a young matchmaker, too. I often coordinated the set-up teams and put people I knew liked each other together to work on a project - so they got to know each other.

When I was in my sophomore year of high school, my parents permitted a friend to come and live with us because her parents were going through a nasty divorce, and she often got caught up in the crossfire. They eventually got divorced, and she moved in with her mom. It felt so good to help her out – with a beautiful ending.

Early Career, Friendships & Growing

Upon graduating from high school, I worked for a restaurant and a pharmacy and, on the weekends, for a caterer, mostly doing corporate events and weddings. I loved this combination of activities, and every day was an adventure. I quickly learned the ropes of excellent event planning and was offered an internship at a prestigious law firm. This is where my skills in event planning, people management, and learning about cultural diversity gave me a love of people, places, and adventurers.

I was the "go-to person at the firm" for fixing emotional meltdowns, keeping things calm, and raising the bar for employee appreciation and affirmations.

Because of this, I often befriended, primarily women, in challenging situations and spent my weekends doing childcare, helping with odd jobs, or just being a friend.

I never thought I was in any way doing anything heroic or special. It wasn't until years later that I realized how many people I impacted that impacted who I became.

The secretary was having an affair with one of the older firm attorneys, and through our relationship (and my matchmaking skills), she found true love outside the office.

There was the young mom who had to work and provide for her 3 other children, and by teaming up with her and some of the other moms, we were able to get the firm to create the first daycare center for working moms inside the firm.

There was the "cultural" appreciation luncheon that I was part of each year, where we all brought in our favorite foods and shared stories of what it was like to be who we were (Black, Brown, Yellow, White - precious in his sight...). We helped each other job share, cover each other's shifts, and cater to each other, and through it all, I grew to appreciate people for where they were and what they could give.

I loved seeing change and growth in those around me and the firm, which became the first to do many things for women and minorities in the corporate world. (First childcare, first job share, first on-the-job training program, first community outreach project) and much more. I had no idea then that this would propel me into working with transformational leaders, coaches, authors, and speakers.

Lasting Love and Family

I met my husband, Memory Dennis, in line at McDonalds. He was handsome and flirty, so after a conversation, I gave him my number (I actually gave him my parents' number). After all, I was young, working in a law firm, and had a hectic schedule, and I knew my mom would properly screen him for me. He was recently divorced, had 2 boys (2 and 4), was a real estate agent, and was a professional water skier.

We met in June, and by the time we had our actual first date (in October), Dennis had gone to Sunday dinners, golf outings, and family game nights, and my parents had put pressure on me to have a date with him since they had been dating him for months.

We dated for a couple of years, then he and the boys took me back to the McDonald's where we met, and he put my engagement ring in a Big Mac box, and in unison, they asked me to marry "them."

Being the person I was, I said YES and immediately made dinner with his ex-wife to let her know I was coming aboard. I would never dream of replacing her or interrupting her relationship with the boys.

During these years, 4 other children became our "kids."

When my sister passed away, we took in my 2 nephews (Chris, who was 10, and Robbie, who was 6). They shuttle between our house and the grandparents' home.

Knowing instinctively how important it was for the boys to have relationships with all the family members, I tried to be their voice of reason and champion for their activities, causes, and ability to learn to live without their mom.

During this same time, a dear neighbor friend of ours also passed away, and we took in her 6-year-old (Matthew). Matthew and Robbie shared a room, and we fondly called them brothers from different mothers whom we loved unconditionally. All 3 of these boys (my 2 nephews and our friend's boy) lost their moms at a very young age. My nephews eventually lost their father, as he passed away at a young age, and Matt never knew his dad. So, Dennis and I became "all their mom & dad."

It has been my privilege to guide these 5 boys through dating, education, discovering who they are, and watching them become wonderful humans.

But our story continues. When Matt was 17 ½, he had to do a family tree project on ancestry for school, so he went to find some of his other family members and came home and said his niece would be going into foster care and could do something. So, we met with the social workers, got the parents to sign off and give us custody, and this is how we got our daughter, Nina! Nina came to stay with us when she was 8 years old. We had the most fun with her. After raising 5 boys, having a strong female influence in the home was excellent.

I have been so blessed to have the gift of being the mom to these 6 amazing people. Here is a little summary of how proud we are:

DJ is the eldest. He is married with 4 children. 1 of his boys recently married and gave us all our first great-grandson. He grew up playing bagpipes, loves his Scottish heritage, and is the family politician.

Ryan is next. He is married with 2 children. He's our artist and electrician by trade. Loving and giving heart - he will be there for you through thick and thin.

Then comes Chris, who is single and lives with us. He is gifted and a great composer of music and loves to edit videos.

Next is Robbie. Married with 2 children. He's our profound thinker, likes order, loves the military, and works in loss prevention.

Then there is Matthew. He is married with 2 children. He's our dreamer and educator and loves being around family and community. He coaches soccer, is a teacher, and is the first in his family to graduate with honors.

Last, but not least, is Nina. Single. In college and stepping into management at Starbucks. She keeps Dennis in coffee and me in stories of the many people she meets.

All our kids have worked with me at events and have been subjected to the wonderful world of entrepreneurship. Each of them, in their own way, has contributed to making my business better. They are the reason I do my work and give so much to my clients. Our journey together spanned four decades of a solid and loving marriage. If you were counting above, I have 6 kids, 10 grandkids, and 1 great-grandson! This crew all started early – meaning tons more time to plan adventures together.

The Heart and Soul of Blu Diamond Events

At Blu Diamond Event Management, we approach events with a unique perspective – one driven by focusing on solutions. After all, raising 6 kids will keep you on your toes, and when it comes to helping clients, hardly anything gets done past me. I've learned to think ahead, examine situations, and dig deep to pull out the truths, dreams, hidden goals, and gems inside my clients. I've seen it all, felt it all, and experienced it all. Being calm for our clients while handling all the details is the heart and soul of Blu Diamond.

An event is not just about numbers on a balance sheet; it's about creating meaningful connections, leaving a lasting impact on attendees, and nurturing relationships with our clients while building communities. We don't just plan parties; we create human experiences, connections, and magical life-changing moments.

God has graciously gifted me with an impressive client list, wonderful children, a loving family, a devoted husband, and some of the best friends and clients in the world.

Through the work my team and I do in the event planning space, we have created extraordinary lifestyles for our clients and our families and have incorporated the love of country, community, and the appreciation for different cultures around the world into who we are.

My journey as an event planner has revealed the immense power of compassion and transformation within my soul. I have seen firsthand how a well-crafted event can create positive, long-lasting change in businesses and individuals' lives. I live for those goosebumps moments when an event transcends the ordinary and becomes extraordinary. Through creativity, thought leadership, and out-of-the-box thinking, we craft experiences that inspire personal growth and empower attendees to reach new heights.

The heartwarming stories shared by those who have attended our events speak volumes about our impact. Witnessing lives change and transformations happen at events is the most rewarding aspect of my career. It reaffirms my belief in the power within each person to shape their destiny and achieve greatness.

Conclusion

As I reflect on my journey as a visionary event planner and the journey of love and resilience in my personal life, I am humbled and inspired. At the "heart" of it all, I believe in bringing people together and creating human connections - whether for charity fundraisers, corporate conferences, lavish weddings, coaching and business programs, or just a good ol' party. Through our event-driven business model, we have helped clients generate millions in revenue from repeatable events.

"The Powerful She" is not just about me; it's a celebration of every individual's potential to make a difference in the world. Through integrity, authenticity, and the relentless pursuit of excellence, I have channeled my passion for events to touch the lives of many.

This chapter has been a heartfelt exploration of my professional achievements, love for events, and the profound impact of family and compassion in shaping my character. I hope my story inspires others to embrace their uniqueness, discover their power within, and create extraordinary experiences that leave a legacy. As I continue my journey, I am grateful for the unwavering support of my family and the opportunities to touch lives and transform the world one event at a time.

Linda Cain

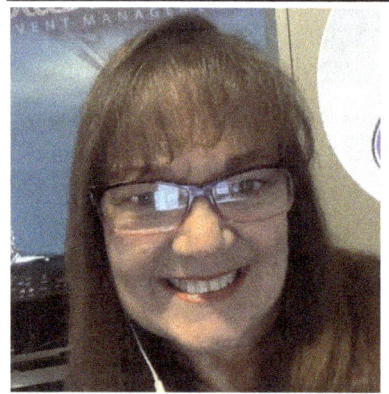

Linda Cain, CEO & Founder of Blu Diamond Events, is all about events. Whether in-person, virtual, hybrid, or high-end destination retreats, Linda and her team at Blu Diamond believe hosting events is the number one way to drive revenue to your business, create lasting relationships and community, and expand your visibility and influence to be purposely impactful. They help their clients map out a 6 & 7 7-figure event-driven Business success plan using events as part of their marketing strategy and focusing on critical activities that will drive revenue, fill their events, and create extraordinary experiences. Linda's diverse background and experience planning domestic and international events for over 25 years have positioned her and her team as the sought-after event producers in the entrepreneurial and coaching industry. Linda and her team are all about the "heart" and "relationship" of events and their clients. With a Rolodex of the "who's who" in the transformational, coaching, and entrepreneur space, this team helps create, plan, and produce consistent 6 & 7-figure events with repeatable processes to maximize profits. Linda's clients love her calmness under pressure and "can do" attitude that drives her whole team and puts her clients at ease. When not planning events, Linda travels with her husband and family, raises Pomeranians, reads, and spends time in peace!

Website: https://www.eventsbybludiamond.com/
Facebook: https://www.facebook.com/linda.cain.3532/
Instagram: https://www.instagram.com/eventsbybludiamond/?hl=en
LinkedIn: https://www.linkedin.com/in/bludiamond

Millions & Minefields
TRAPPED BY EXPECTATION
Tiffany Cui

Born into privilege in the heart of China's Sichuan province, home of pandas and spicy food, I was the only child of a family that exemplified excellence. My grandma is an OBGYN and President of the Women's Hospital; my grandpa is an eye surgeon and military general; my mom is a university professor; and my dad is a family physician. Plus, all our close relatives were in powerful and high-earning positions. They filled my tiny world with love, abundance, elite education, and lofty expectations.

My life had been meticulously charted - premiere schools, a prestigious profession, a marriage of equivalent or higher social status, high-achieving children, a beautiful home, and a retirement befitting our family legacy. However, this well-crafted path took an unexpected turn when I was fourteen, and my mom decided to move our family to the United States. Suddenly, I found myself in an alien world, unable to understand the language, struggling in a completely foreign culture. I was faced with a vast and daunting task - adapt or suffer.

This was quite the learning curve, but I found the strength and flourished, especially growing up in New York City, a mixed language, race, and culture environment. I pursued an education at a prestigious university and secured high-profile jobs in Silicon Valley. I was living the American dream, with a six-figure salary, a lucrative investment property portfolio, traveling the world, and the keys to my then dream house. Yet, despite all these accomplishments, I felt like a walking zombie without purpose or fulfillment. The monotony of the 9-5 grind was like death by a thousand cuts. My soul bled, slowly and constantly.

I found an escape in the biographies of famous and inspiring people and discovered my hero, Coco Chanel. Her journey from the orphanage to becoming a designer, an entrepreneur, living the most fabulous and intriguing life, going through WWII, becoming the world's most famous designer, and a titan in the fashion world whose legacy endures today.

As I navigated my way through over two decades of corporate career, entrepreneurship always held an inexplicable allure. The thrill of unpredictability, constant challenge, and infinite learning opportunities felt like stepping onto a rollercoaster ride that could veer in any direction at any moment. It was intoxicating.

Spurred by this entrepreneurial desire, I plunged headfirst into the world of e-commerce, launching a company that sold jewelry with message cards. While I initially ran the entire operation, eventually, I brought on a business partner who was more experienced in e-commerce, hoping to speed up my learning curve and accelerate growth.

However, my enthusiasm clouded my judgment, leading me into an arrangement where I contributed 100% of the capital while sharing profits 50-50.

The competition was fierce. Despite being carefully curated and uniquely messaged, our products were up against hundreds, if not thousands, of similar sellers. Our strategy was simple yet uncertain:

- Create as many messages as we can.
- Test them through Facebook ads.
- One of them will resonate with our audience and inspire purchases.

We played the numbers game, spending hundreds of thousands of dollars on ad testing, betting on the model "if they cry, they buy."

Against the odds, we struck gold. Holidays became our savior, especially Valentine's Day, Mother's Day, and Father's Day, with personalized jewelry becoming an instant bestseller. We were riding a wave of success, reaching an all-time high of $30K a day and cumulating $1.1 million in our first eighteen months. These numbers were a testament to the grueling long hours, the missed social events, and the countless trials and errors. It was a triumph of dedication, grit, and every moment of sacrifice. Every ounce of effort, every drop of sweat, and every tear shed was worth it.

But with this high, a low was waiting around the corner.

We expanded quickly to a full-time staff of eight and engaged consulting firms to bolster our marketing efforts. However, the profits from our holiday sales vanished, absorbed by payroll and consulting fees. As sales slowed during the summer, the dwindling cash reserves became an unnerving specter that haunted my nights.

To mitigate the crisis, we resorted to loans, an option I initially hesitated about due to my upbringing and cultural aversion to debt. However, the need to keep the company afloat was desperate. The initial small loan I took on was quickly repaid thanks to the success of Father's Day sales. The relief, however, was fleeting.

The slow sales and overhead continued to drain us. We were bleeding cash every day, struggling with the financial burden of an oversized staff, underperforming consulting firms, and increased advertising costs. We took painful measures to slow the outflow, downsizing our staff and terminating all consulting services. But still, the cash flow issue persisted, forcing me to take on two more substantial loans in the hope that Christmas holiday sales would save our business.

The holiday sales were decent but fell short of incredible. I managed to pay off one of the loans but was left grappling with the other six-figure loan and a six-figure credit card debt. My finances were in a state of wreckage. When I approached my business partner to contribute capital, I was shocked by a revelation: he was saddled in debt from a previous failed business.

We were in a deadlock, with no cash reserves or means to generate revenue.

It was clear that my only option was to shut down the company. As I struggled with the reality of the massive debt that I was personally responsible for, I spiraled downward into physical, mental, and emotional distress. The following eight months were a brutal struggle with failure and consequences.

Metamorphosis

A year and a half of grinding 18 hours a day, 7 days a week, began to take its toll on my mind, body, and spirit. I had pushed my limits to the extreme, and finally, my body buckled under exhaustion. Mornings became an insurmountable challenge as I struggled to get out of bed. Once sharp and focused, my mind could barely concentrate for more than ten minutes at a time.

As a Chinese woman, the social expectations imprinted on me since childhood were hard to shake off. Their definition of success as a prestigious job, a high social standing, a hefty bank balance, and a picture-perfect family felt like a phantom that had haunted me throughout life. At that moment, every metric that could be used to measure my success was showing my failure. I was jobless, in debt, with a failed business, and now I was at risk of losing my home.

My shame was so overwhelming that I withdrew and isolated myself from my loved ones. I shrank away from family gatherings and hid my shame. I judged myself harshly, labeling myself as a monumental Failure. Yes, failure with a capital "F." Every glance in the mirror reflected an individual I no longer recognized, someone who had failed everyone around her—my parents, my family, the love of my life, and above all, myself.

One day, while driving, the emotional dam I had constructed against my pain finally broke. The tears poured down my face, mirroring the rivers of self-loathing and regret that had swallowed me. I felt my fingernails digging into my thigh; each indent a silent scream of my suffering. Then, I stopped at a light, my other hand let go of the steering wheel, formed a fist, and started punching myself in the head. The self-inflicted pain, instead of offering an escape, drove me further into my darkness. My man, my love, witnessing my anguish, was shocked and heartbroken to see me this way. He pulled me out of my self-destructive trance; his calm strength in the face of my turmoil was the rock and pillar of strength I needed, my life raft in the tumultuous sea of my despair.

The next day, as I stood under the shower, the remnants of the pain from my self-inflicted wounds served as a stark reminder of my mental and emotional torment. My world seemed to narrow to one question: "Where do I go from here?" Should I accept defeat and wither away, or was another path waiting for me? The title of failure I generously bestowed upon myself clung to me like a stain.

In this darkness, I found solace in books and podcasts. Works like The Untethered Soul, The Obstacle is The Way, Becoming, Breaking the Habit of Being Yourself, Super Soul (podcast), and others became my guiding stars. Through their wisdom, I began to see the darkness as a necessary precursor to the dawn of new insight. As Eckhart Tolle's words echoed in my mind:

"The dark night of the soul is a kind of death that you die. What dies is the egoic sense of self. Of course, death is always painful, but nothing real has died there – only an illusory identity. It's a kind of re-birth, is part of the awakening process, the death of the old self and the birth of the true self." Once you have been re-born, you will *"look upon events, people, and so on with a deep sense of aliveness, sense the aliveness through your sense of aliveness, but you are not trying to fit your experience into a conceptual framework anymore."*

I started to see the path to step out of my predetermined social expectations and create a new vision that aligns with my desires and aspirations.

The silver lining in this turmoil was the unwavering support of my man. A true visionary is a leader with the gift of vision - the ability to see what others can't, in themselves and in life. And - in me. He could see my journey and experiences as life's hard lessons in the "School of Hard Knocks" rather than a failure. He shined the light that became my beacon of hope. He saw my strength, courage, and dedication, showing me that a single failed venture did not define me. His tireless support and the wisdom and self-awareness I gained during this dark period readied me for the next chapter in my life.

Slowly, my heart lightened. With newfound vision and focus, I dusted off the last few remnants of anguish and despair and eagerly looked forward to new adventures.

From Darkness to Direction

From the darkness of my entrepreneurial heartbreak emerged a profound clarity. Sometimes, our greatest challenges become our brightest beacons of purpose. Just like Coco Chanel transformed her humble beginnings into an empire built on vision and determination, my journey through the shadows revealed my true calling: guiding others to find their light.

Daily Vision was co-founded during this transformative experience with my greatest supporter, who saw my potential even in my darkest moments. Together, we created a space for leaders seeking to transform their personal and professional challenges into stepping stones toward visionary leadership.

The same resilience that pulled me through my entrepreneurial crisis now fuels my passion for nurturing and empowering women in leadership roles. Every tear shed, every moment of doubt, and every hard-won lesson has become a lantern I can hold up for others navigating their own challenging paths. Through Daily Vision, we illuminate the way forward with emotional intelligence, character-driven leadership, and strategic vision.

My journey taught me that true leadership isn't just about seeing the path ahead. It's about helping others find their way through the fog of uncertainty. When I work with executives and entrepreneurs today, I share not just strategies and frameworks but the deep understanding that our greatest struggles often precede our most meaningful transformations. This isn't just business coaching; it's about awakening the visionary within each leader we touch.

As Eckhart Tolle's wisdom about the "dark night of the soul" resonated during my transformation, it now echoes in the corridors of our coaching practice. We guide our clients to embrace their challenges as catalysts for growth, helping them emerge stronger, more authentic, and better equipped to lead with vision and purpose.

The choice to rise from adversity still presents itself every day, but now I help others make that choice, too. Through Daily Vision, we're creating a legacy of leaders who understand that character, integrity, and self-awareness are the foundations of visionary leadership. Every leader we empower becomes a beacon of hope and guidance for others, creating a ripple effect of positive transformation in the business world.

Author G. Michael Hopf's words about hard times creating strong individuals ring truer than ever. These challenges don't just test us; they awaken something profound within us. A strength that transforms not only our own lives but touches the lives of others. Embrace your story, embrace your strength, embrace your purpose.

Tiffany Cui

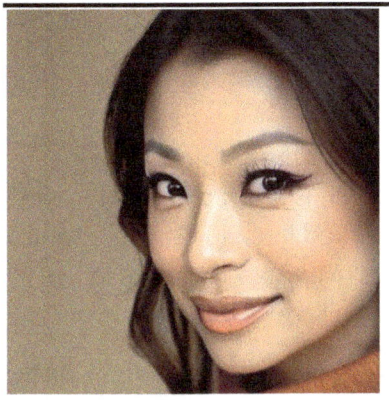

Tiffany Cui is a leadership coach specializing in helping women in leadership roles get results. She is a co-author of the book The Powerful She and the co-founder of DAILY VISION Executive Coaching.

Tiffany's career spans more than twenty years in business, accounting, and finance. She spearheaded compliance for Gap, Inc. in San Francisco, risk management and governance for Boyd Gaming in Las Vegas, and international expansion for Sierra Asia Partners in the U.S. and China. She owned and operated a boutique accounting firm in San Francisco, renovated and resold over thirty homes in Las Vegas, created a 7-figure e-commerce jewelry store, and contributed to The Powerful She with transformational leadership lessons for women empowering women.

Tiffany is passionate about nurturing and empowering women in leadership roles. Her mission is to guide them in their visionary leadership and equip them with the skills and tools to create meaningful results.

Facebook: https://www.facebook.com/tiffany.cui.3
Instagram: https://www.instagram.com/tiffanylcui/
LinkedIn: http://www.linkedin.com/in/tiffany-cui-daily-vision

The Unveiling
Carl-a Diran

My name is Carla Diran, and I am a mother of a wonderful, dynamic 8-year-old child. I work as a child therapist and a board-certified behavior analyst. I have worked in child development, specifically autism, for over 20 years. My road to get here was difficult, but details of my struggles will come later.

I always believed that a person's life story begins before birth. Our culture, ancestry, and especially our family of origin are unavoidable and essential parts of our life. My story starts back in Istanbul, Turkey, in 1915. My great-grandfather was the founder of the first Armenian Masonic Lodge in Turkey. He was a 33rd-degree mason and revered by many. He had 5 children (one boy and 4 girls). My grandfather was the oldest and the first of our family to finish high school. At 18, my grandfather left to work for a shipping company outside of London. Sadly, he didn't know this would be the last time he saw his mother and two of his four sisters alive. The genocide happened while he was away. My great-grandfather was barely able to escape with two of his daughters, while sadly, his wife and two other girls were murdered. I remember my father telling me this story as a young girl. He said all your grandfather got from his father was a telegram, which said in Armenian, "Keep going."

Leaving Homeland

My grandfather knew precisely what this meant. So, he never went back home again. Instead, he moved to France, where he lived a good life in Marseilles and worked for a shipping company. He was only 25 and fluent in Turkish, Russian, French, English, and Armenian. After a while, he was sent on a mission to Romania and fell in love with the country. He met my grandmother in Bucharest one day; it was love at first sight. The two had three children (a boy and 2 girls). My father was the oldest of the three. My grandfather became very wealthy, and the family had a gorgeous apartment in the city and a lovely country home. Once again, tragedy hit World War II. In 1945 when the Nazis were defeated, the Russians came in and took everything away. My father's family was now destitute. They lived poor and meek lives, as did most Romanians and Eastern Europeans then.

Time moved on, and my father was a horrible student and a significant troublemaker, so much so that his parents sent him to study religion for a year in Moscow. This experience scared him so severely that he returned home from Russia and began attending school and getting good grades. Once he graduated high school, he was so afraid to go into the army (which was required by all unless you were accepted into a university) that one summer, he locked himself in a tiny attic room and did nothing but study. When it came time to take a test to get into the university, his grades were the highest of roughly 4,000 others.

A New Life

Soon after, he met my mother. She was a troubled and poor girl (6 years his junior). They, too, instantly fell in love. But her dark past would eventually lead to a relationship so toxic it almost destroyed my life. But that's to come at a later time. My mother's mother had my mother at 16. She had been raped by a 32-year-old man whom she was forced to marry and who physically and mentally abused her. When my mother was 3 years old, my grandmother divorced my grandfather and gave my mom up to her brother and his wife. She had not seen my mother for 3 years. During that time, my grandmother met another man and had another daughter. They, too, divorced, and my half-aunt was taken from my grandmother. Desperate to get my mother back, she reclaimed her from her brother. The two of them developed a very sick-meshed relationship that lasts to this day.

In 1970, my father was allowed to leave Romania because of his Armenian heritage and immigrate to the USA. He went with his parents and one of his sisters. They had nothing. They had to live in Lebanon in disgusting conditions, not knowing the language, and getting by with my grandfather's wits and ability to speak French. Imagine one tiny room with no heat and no AC. The four of them would live off one chicken for an entire week. Finally, six months later, they arrived in New York. My father's other sister was in Los Angeles and offered to help them once they got to LA, but they needed to spend one night in NYC. Once again, they were placed in a seedy motel in a horrible part of the city. My father woke up with roaches all over him that night. Then, he swore he would never be poor or hungry again.

The next day, they arrived in LA. My father's brother-in-law did all he could to help my father get a job. They lived in an apartment that was part of a building my uncle was able to buy. My father worked as a bookkeeper at a company that bought and sold glass jars and bottles. He saved until he could buy a car and bring my mother to the United States after he married her in Romania. She got a job working for a CPA firm, and they were eventually able to buy a little house. A year later, my mother's mother also came to Los Angeles. This was the beginning of the end. They began to fight constantly because my mother was always siding with my grandmother, and soon, they were fighting every day.

My mother had had five abortions before she found out she was pregnant with me. For whatever reason ordained by God, she told my father, "I want to keep this one." And so, I was born. My father was ecstatic. From what I was told, I was his golden child. He immediately tried to make things work with my mother, but she was always unhappy, cold, and neglectful. I know this is a fact because that's exactly how she was towards me. My maternal grandmother and my father raised me. I had never known my father's mother, as she passed away from cancer before I was born. My earliest memories are only those of my parents yelling and screaming when they thought I was asleep. Fortunately, some good ones were my grandmother taking me for stroller rides and my dad taking me to the park. But the yelling was always there. I felt it was my fault.

The Love (not)

Then, in my young life (as far as I am concerned), tragedy struck. Imagine one day waking up to my step-grandfather watching me, and my mom, dad, and grandma are all gone. I was 3 ½ years old. He wouldn't tell me where they were, only that my aunt would pick me up after work. He then touched me in ways I did not know what to do. He claimed it was love. I knew it was wrong. I wanted to scream, but no one was there, so I waited for my aunt. When she picked me up, I remember feeling so relieved. I never told her or anyone else what had happened.

Two days later, my parents and grandmother came home. But they weren't alone. Nope. They had something small with them. I now apparently had a sister. No one had warned me, nor did I understand the concept. My mother doted on her day and night—something I never had. My mother would shove me away when I would get close to maybe getting a hug. I developed a hatred for this new being, thinking she was some pet. Through all this, my father worked hard to build his successful business, and my mother became a CPA. All the while, the fighting continued every night. I remember putting my hands over my sister's ears so she would not hear what I had been hearing since I was born.

As time passed, my parents separated, and we moved into quite a large home. They slept in different bedrooms, and the fighting subsided somewhat. In the meantime, I was constantly pulling pranks on my sister and having fights with her. Both my parents were sick of it and would side with her. Of course, I know now that I was inadvertently doing it intentionally and for attention (mainly from my mother). But throughout these times, something powerful was growing in me. A strength that I did not recognize was there until I was 7 years old.

Finding My Inner Strength

While driving to our condo in Palm Springs, I started yet another fight with my sister. My father got so mad that he turned and told me that if I didn't stop it right there and then, he'd leave me on the side of the freeway. And he did just that. He stopped the car and asked me to step out. Thinking I would run back to the car, I decided to walk the other way. It was then and there that I knew I had had enough.

Despite the early childhood trauma that I endured with neglect and abuse; I carried on quite well in school academically. Socially, however, this was a completely different story. I was raised only with Romanian food and rarely ate burgers or chicken nuggets. I would be dressed in a European style, as my mother would take us to Europe every year for vacation. I was laughed at and made fun of...kind of like the girl in "My Big Fat Greek Wedding." Then, to add insult to injury, I was moved to another private school in 8th grade. That was even worse as the kids had already formed "clicks." I would eat my lunch in bathroom stalls and stay away from others as much as possible. Instead, I studied hard and focused on academics. At least, that's one thing my parents agreed on. Education.

At 10 years old, tragedy struck again when my father came home and said he was leaving us. My life was never the same. My mother had filed a restraining order against him and filed for divorce. He told me that my life was over and that no one would love a girl whose parents were divorced. Something shattered within me as a young girl full of hopes and dreams. But it did not deter me, as will later be seen.

Found Grace

The divorce was a long and terrifying one. I was in the middle of their tug-of-war. Each one says, "They hate the other more than they love me." It was then that I started seeing a court-appointed psychologist. Let me tell you, this woman changed my world. She made me feel safe and calm. She gave me strength and hope. But most of all, she gave me (then) an identity that was mine.

I learned I did not need to please anyone anymore. I just needed to be myself. This woman made me decide, without a doubt, that my life's mission is to help and work with children. Since I never wandered from this path. I graduated high school with honors and went to university to study two of my passions, psychology and French.

The internal struggle didn't end, though. I still had very low self-esteem and was easily hurt by others. Their opinion always meant so much to me. Although I was excelling academically and socially, I was struggling. So, I joined a sorority. I made several great friends, and we partied like most kids do in college. But my friend and I were similar. We both weren't the sorority kind. So, we left the sorority and moved in together. I changed my hair color, started dressing way more fashionably, did a lot of shopping, and traveled whenever possible. Despite all this, I found one boyfriend, and low and behold, he was abusive and more emotional. He'd constantly tell me how to dress (which was not my style) and always call me fat (which, in retrospect, I was not).

By 21, I had broken up with him, but not without repercussion. I had developed anorexia and would eat about 300 calories a day. When we broke up, I was 5'3" and weighed 98 pounds. That's when my mother (for the first time) intervened and took me to see a psychologist. I was placed on anti-depressants and, within a year, had gained a considerable amount of weight. Nevertheless, the one thing that didn't falter within me was my studies and my work.

I met Dr. Lovass (a founder in applied behavior analysis) and fell in love with the subject. I knew from his classes and from interning with him that this would be my life's path: working with children with autism and developmental and emotional disorders. Even though things seemed to be in a good place, things changed once again.

In grad school, I met a man online. He was visiting his father, who lived in San Diego. We instantly fell in love. I had never felt so loved before. We moved into my place rather quickly. My parents were against him because he wasn't working. We were together for two years before we got married - without my father's consent. This was culturally huge, but I always did what I felt was right because of the inner strength I found within me. A few months later, I was pregnant. Sadly, I was threatened with either having an abortion or losing my inheritance.

My respect for my father was tremendous, and I gave in. It wasn't long before we divorced at my father's will but decided to move away to Vienna together. There, I got my second master's degree in international relations and began to find myself again. Sadly, the abortion took its toll on him, and we split up. I had no choice but to live alone in Vienna, where I taught psychologists and psychiatrists and became a therapist for applied behavior analysis.

I felt I mattered for the first time and wanted to stay and evolve.

Years later, I returned home to Los Angeles. I worked my way up from being a one-on-one therapist to owning my own company and now as a regional clinical director for a major company in California.

The road has been challenging. Even though work has always been excellent, at 33, I felt like my love life was over for me. I thought I would never remarry or have a child.

My True Love - In Early 2013, I met the love of my life. We got engaged and married, and together, we have this fantastic 9-year-old who is thriving and wants to follow in her mama's footsteps when she grows up.

I am and feel truly blessed. All my trials and tribulations, which led to success, help you know that everything and anything is possible to achieve when there's the will, the drive, and the passion.

Never falter from your dreams – they do become a reality!

Carla Diran

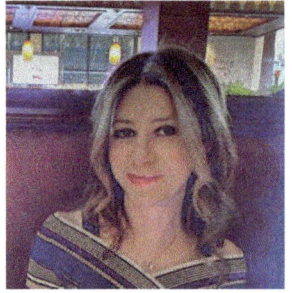

Carla Diran MA BCBA. Carla is a board-certified behavior analyst working with children with autism and other related disorders for 20 years. She is highly trained in developing children's skill sets to help them mainstream in society and function without being labeled. Carla firmly believes in parent training, helping parents understand their child's condition, and helping them use strategies and methods to create a consistent and natural growing and healing environment for their children.

As a behavioral analyst working with autistic children, Carla's role is crucial in helping these children develop the necessary skills and behaviors to improve their quality of life and social interactions. Her primary objective is to assess and analyze the child's behavior, identify areas of difficulty or challenges, and develop effective intervention plans to address those specific needs.

Her work as a behavioral analyst can profoundly impact the lives of these children and their families. She approaches her role with compassion, dedication, and a commitment to helping each child reach their full potential.

Facebook: https://www.facebook.com/carla.diran
LinkedIn: https://www.linkedin.com/in/carla-diran-1089a722

Resilience Unleashed
A WOMAN'S RISE TO EMPOWERMENT
Lady Jen Du Plessis

Reflecting on my journey, I'm reminded that transformation is not a singular event but an ongoing evolution. The path I've walked, marked by twists and turns, has led me to a place where the limitations of my past no longer define me. This chapter encapsulates my narrative, struggles, and triumphs—a testament to the power of resilience, self-discovery, and personal growth.

Breaking Through Barriers: A Glimpse into My Past

Growing up, my story was shaped by a tapestry of challenges. I am the daughter of an alcoholic father and a verbally abusive mother. In an environment where demonstrating love was scarce and acceptance felt unattainable, I struggled with self-confidence from an early age. The echoes of hurtful words reverberated in my mind, breeding self-doubt and inhibiting my ability to embrace my potential. It's in these early experiences that the seeds of my journey were planted. My family nicknamed me "Jenny, who ain't got a penny," which marked years of turbulence and uncertainty, wondering if I could ever be enough.

In my early career, these scars followed me, manifesting as self-doubt and a yearning for validation. My career path wasn't immune to the wounds of my past. Despite my achievements, I grappled with a relentless sense of inadequacy. The fear of not measuring up, of not being enough, cast a shadow on my accomplishments. The whispers of my past became a barrier I had to break through—one that required an unwavering commitment to self-discovery and healing. Despite my accomplishments, a cloud of self-criticism loomed over me, clouding my vision and preventing me from fully embracing my potential.

Throughout my career, I embraced opportunities to learn and grow, even in the face of skepticism. Each obstacle I overcame, each glass ceiling I shattered, added another layer to my power. But true power isn't about conquest but lifting others as we rise. Mentorship became my calling as I realized that sharing my journey could inspire and empower those who walked similar paths.

Yet, as the years rolled on, something shifted within me. At 48, I stood at a crossroads, confronted with a choice: to let my past define me or rise above it. With unwavering determination, I embarked on a journey of self-discovery and healing. It was a path paved with moments of introspection, difficult conversations, and a commitment to rewrite the narrative I had internalized for far too long.

So many years of wasting time, energy, and life while chasing the dreams of others, believing they were dreams I wanted too. I was at a so-called "diner" with my family one night when I received a phone call from a client. Of course, I took the call! – my client needed me. While outside the restaurant talking to the client and walking on what I now refer to as the "concrete balance beam," aka the curb, I happened to look over into the restaurant window. There they were, my family, laughing, joking, playing with straws and water – creating beautiful memories. Memories that I wouldn't be in yet again because I was too wrapped up in my mission of proving to everyone that I could be more than what everyone thought -Jenny who ain't got a penny" – the little girl who would grow up to be nothing- worthless – poor – an alcoholic.

At that moment, I decided I was done proving myself and would start living life the way I wanted, not some dream someone else had for me. I remember my mentor, Les Brown, saying, "If you are casual about your dreams, your dreams will become a casualty." It was time to live with the utmost intention, and I learned that intention is *everything*!

As so it happened, that love became the foundation of my transformation, becoming my healing relief. I learned to love myself, my imperfections, and all. This self-love was a rebellion against the voices that once told me I wasn't enough. It reminded me that I deserved the love and compassion I had always sought.

Love, Grace, and Courage: The Catalysts for Removing My Shell and Becoming Authentic

For the next several years, I worked on myself daily. I broke through so many barriers and limiting beliefs. Ultimately creating "a work life that made life work." I had cracked the code on integrating life and work without sacrificing either. I learned the art of exuding happiness in all endeavors.

The triumvirate of love, grace, and courage is at the core of my transformation. Love became my foundation—a force that empowered me to dismantle the walls I had built around my heart. I learned to love myself, acknowledging that my imperfections were not flaws to hide but facets to embrace. This self-love was an act of defiance against the self-critical voices that had held me captive for far too long.

Grace, a virtue I had underestimated, was pivotal in my growth. Extending grace to my parents, recognizing that their struggles were not a reflection of my worth, was a transformative step. Forgiving them was an act of liberation—a release from the chains of resentment that had bound me to the past.

In the face of self-doubt, courage emerged as my guiding light. It took courage to confront my past, to unravel the layers of self-criticism, and to step into leadership roles I once believed were beyond my reach. This daily act of courage reshaped my narrative, allowing me to replace insecurity with empowerment. I was living in abundance rather than scarcity, a concept I failed to comprehend in my earlier years. I remember telling business associates that I didn't need any help; I was "good," "okay," and "can handle it." Later, I learned that I was merely hiding the fact that I lacked self-confidence and didn't want to show any weakness. All the while, inside, I was screaming for help!

Courage emerged as my guiding light. It took courage to confront my past and release its grip on my present. It took courage to step into leadership roles, to believe that my voice was valuable, and to inspire others through my journey. It was a daily act of courage to silence the self-critical voices and replace them with affirmations of strength.

With each challenge, I've overcome and each barrier I've shattered, I've taken a step closer to becoming the woman I aspire to be. My background, far from limiting me, has fortified my spirit. The resilience I cultivated in the face of adversity became the bedrock of my strength. From my parents' struggles, I drew the determination to carve a different path.

Becoming a Cut Above: Embracing Personal Growth for Massive Success

Nearing 60, I stand as living proof that the journey to empowerment is a continuous evolution. From the scars of my past, I have emerged as a woman who refuses to be defined by her history. The phrase "a cut above" resonates deeply with me—a reminder that I am no longer bound by the person I used to be. I realized that I could be myself; everyone else was already taken. Being myself isn't bad at all; in fact, I like – no - love myself exactly as I am (even with my flaws!).

This journey has been extended, yet it is very rewarding. Having been in the mortgage and financial industry for 4 decades, and as a token woman in the early years, through tenacity and toughness really, I became a pioneer, a veteran, and an icon for other women to achieve their goals and dreams in a shorter period. Not only did I break barriers for annual production – landing in the top 200 nationwide mortgage loan originators (from a pool of 785,000)- but I accomplished this five times in my career. Then there was the concluding production task of closing over $1 Billion in mortgage loans – this feat less than 50 people have done in history. Several other achievements, honors, and awards were bestowed over those and subsequent years, amassing to my most recent honor of being Knighted as a *Dame* by the Royal House of Cappadocia of the Holy Roman Empire of the East, into the Royal Order of Constantine the Great and Saint Helen.

Me? *Lady Jen Du Plessis*. From such a humble beginning, struggles, prejudices, awakenings, power, calm, love, courage, fulfillment, happiness, and giving, to becoming a dedicated and loving wife, fantastic mother and grandmother, brilliant businesswoman, caring friend, devoted Christian, supportive volunteer in numerous charitable works, and making an impact in others' lives, while creating significance and leaving *my* mark in this world.

I'm so excited for what lies ahead in my life, God willing, a long life. Now that I am awakened and present in all I do, I can't imagine what God has in store for this life of purpose, achievement, love, and devotion. I only know that I'm ready! I'm much more robust and prepared to take anything on, with tenacity and resilience like never before. So, go ahead, 'Tell me I Can't,' and watch me soar!

My journey is about breaking through barriers and dismantling the walls I had unwittingly built within myself. Delving into my story, allow others to witness the journey of a woman who refused to be defined by her past, who chose to turn her wounds into wellsprings of wisdom, and who is living her legacy while she continues to build it. One who dares others to "tell me I can't, and then get out of my way!"

I've never been a believer in the word empowerment. Whenever I heard someone mention that they 'empower women,' my first thought had been that women must be weak and need someone to help them. That they can't do it alone. Today, I have a different perspective. While I'm still not an absolute fan, I've learned that while living in scarcity, I was not empowered. I was powerful yet hadn't discovered it within myself. Empowerment is an inside job! No one can give you affirmations to quote, meditations to follow, or 'coach' you through it. You are the catalyst for your empowerment, assuming you want it badly enough to create change and become vulnerable to allow others to guide and counsel you through your journey.

I hope that you will see your struggles mirrored in my journey. You will find solace in knowing it's always possible to rewrite your stories, heal old wounds, and step into your power. Through my experiences, you will learn that self-confidence can be reclaimed, that acceptance begins within, and that the path to becoming a mighty woman is marked by love, grace, and courage—qualities that reside within us all, waiting to be awakened.

Inspiration for Your Journey: A Call to Action

As you read my story, I invite you to reflect on your journey. Recognize the barriers you've faced and the strengths you've developed. Embrace the idea that personal growth is not a destination but a life-long journey.

1. **Set Intention:** Identify an area where you can challenge yourself. Write down your intentions and commit to taking tangible steps toward growth.

2. **Practice Self-Compassion:** Extend the same compassion to yourself that you offer to others. Embrace your imperfections as integral parts of your journey.

3. **Embrace Vulnerability:** Share your struggles with someone you trust. Vulnerability fosters connection and growth as you discover you're not alone.

4. **Seek Inspiration:** Surround yourself with stories of resilience and empowerment. Seek out books, podcasts, or online communities that inspire your journey.

5. **Lift Others Along the Way:** As you rise, lift others with you. Mentorship and support have a ripple effect, creating an empowered community.

Remember, your journey is uniquely yours. Embrace your past, celebrate your progress, and continue pushing the boundaries of who you can become. Your potential knows no limits—let your story continue to unfold with courage and conviction.

My journey from self-doubt to empowerment is a testament to the transformation that can occur when we choose to rewrite our narratives. It explores how love, grace, and courage can be harnessed to break through barriers and become a cut above the person we used to be.

Lady Jen Du Plessis

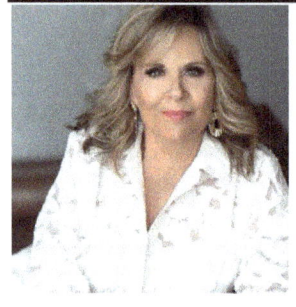

Lady Jen Du Plessis Who would have ever thought that little "Jenny Who Ain't Got a Penny," now Dame Lady Jen, a member of the Royal House of Cappadocia and the Royal Order of Constantine the Great and Saint Helen, would be a charismatic and award-winning international speaker who brings her stories of sorrow, resilience, tenacity, and triumph to every stage she speaks. With numerous #1 best-selling books, hostess of 3 top ranking podcasts, and producer and hostess of her TV show *Business on the Vine*, Lady Jen is certainly making her impact in the world.

Best known as The Team-Building & Scaling Architect, she is the Leading Expert in helping high-achieving business owners and executives build world-class teams live the business lifestyle they always dreamed of to obtain high-performance, tangible outcomes. Her recent awards include the 2024 Impact Mentor of the Year through the International Association of Top Professionals, the 2024 SheLeads Women of Excellence Award, and the 2023 Network of Outstanding Women Mentor of the Year. She received the eZway Network Golden Gala Award for her heart-centered work in the world, as well as the Outstanding Leadership Recognition Award from The Los Angeles Tribune.

She is devoted to her philanthropy and charity work, helping women and children, the homeless, eradicating human trafficking, U.S. Veterans, and Animal Shelters. Lady Jen believes we have Acres of Diamonds right under our feet to inspire people and leave our mark in this world--her motto is "move from working IN and ON your business to living ABOVE and BEYOND."

Website: https://www.jenduplessis.com/
Facebook: https://www.facebook.com/JenDuPlessis22/
Instagram: https://www.instagram.com/jenduplessis/

My Journey into Futures

Manoushag (May) Emirzian

My Journey into Futures. It sounds like a science fiction venture, similar to that of Michael J. Fox and Christopher Lloyd in the 80's film *Back to the Future*. But the type of future I'm referring to has nothing to do with a time machine. I am, in fact, speaking of financial futures, where a trader speculates on an underlying asset's price movement or financial index. If the trader's decision to buy or sell futures is correct, then profit is realized.

It sounds simple. But there are many moving parts, and the path to a successful outcome is only sometimes straight. After all, there is a 50% chance of profit between buying and selling. And profit margins can vary widely.

Realizing the opportunities offered in the market interested me years ago. But the biggest question was: where do I begin?

I researched the subject online and found many educational resources offering complete beginners, intermediate, and advanced courses. Narrowing down these resources requires extensive research of its own. I had to consider the affordability of the course fees, the timeframe to complete these courses, and the accountability of the educator. Even then, after narrowing down my course options, it still felt like a shot in the dark when I "took the plunge" with a course. The curriculum entailed going forward at my own pace, estimating between 3-6 months for completion. However, my excitement about this new venture helped me complete the course in 3 months.

The course shed some light on the probability of market movement, which ultimately helped me decide whether I should buy or sell. I learned about prioritizing profit and loss management and how many contracts to execute. I practiced utilizing tools, such as technical indicators, to help visualize a trend and fundamental indicators, which consider the news and positive or negative changes in previous rates. One example would be a change in the unemployment rate of an earlier report.

So far, the venture is still in discovery— I aim to achieve a reality where I'm ready to trade. However, much education, practice, and testing are needed before involvement in the real financial market. So, I researched platforms that would allow me to practice my skills.

I chose the "Ninja Trader" platform. This platform offered additional classes that familiarized me with researching indicators, giving me the confidence to receive actual data and practice on a simulation account. I also investigated what instrument to trade on commodities, indexes, or Bonds.

Consider the dollar value of each point on a different instrument:

An example would be each point/tick for

Gold = $10.00 - Micro = $1.00

Crude Oil = $10.00 - Micro $1.00

E-Mini S&P = $12.50 - Micro $1.25

Euro = $6.25 - Micro $1.25

Nasdaq = $5.00 - Micro $.50

Ultra Bond = $31.25

I came across many educators in the field. Each had a niche system, claiming their tactic worked most of the time. But I had to ask myself: which approach "fits" my plan? There are many factors to consider. For example, am I prepared for day trading, which involves executing several times in one day? Or am I more suited to swing trading, which entails carrying the trade for more than a day? What is the investment dollar amount one must start with? What trading instrument should I choose? These are all vital questions one must consider before becoming a serious trader.

When considering an investment amount, the simple answer is to start with an amount you can afford to lose. I kept hearing over and over that today's established trading experts lost many times before they became qualified traders, and bit by bit, they improved their strategy.

The more I trade, switching back and forth from simulation to the real market, the more I realize the complexity of trading. I need to look for a strategy to perform at least better than 50%. I need a plan to set the loss to a minimum. I must stick to risk and loss management and target the gain with a much better outcome, adding to a positive overall performance.

I pretty much simplified the process. But why am I struggling to achieve the outcome that I set in mind? Why is my performance inconsistent? I started doubting my ability to be in this venture. These emotions overwhelmed me and forced me to take a recess from trading periodically.

It turns out I'm not alone in this pool of doubt. Statistically speaking, 95% of traders eventually give up due to a lack of success. Part of the reason for such a high quit rate is because of trading competition alongside massive institutions, such as banks. Individual traders like me are constantly trading alongside these big institutions, and guess who has the upper hand? Futures trading is not for the faint of heart.

It became apparent that trading successfully is more than strategy, planning, and setups.

I need to treat my trading as a business I love, not focus only on numbers. To transform my engagement into a pleasant venture, I need to proceed with confidence, focus, and trust in my decisions.

How did I find myself here? Was it an attraction to the financial arena, where there is monetary gain? Was it a spark of curiosity that prompted me to dig further? Was it a mental challenge? Or was my persistence playing a vital role in overcoming the overall difficulties in life?

The first time I heard about trading was through an advertisement offering free training on Forex trading, offering free training. My curiosity moved me to take the classes offered. After some simulation trading, I opened an account and started trading.

At that time, I didn't realize how far I was from mastering many facades of trading, decisions that involve:

- What instrument to trade
- The timeframe to trade in
- How many contracts to trade
- Anticipating the direction of the market
- Overcoming doubts about the decision made
- Being patient and decerning the signals in the market
- Holding good moves in the gain, yet knowing when to exit
- Exiting the market in the event of a downturn
- Managing the account by treating it as a business
- Building confidence with practice.

I discovered that each challenge is a complex issue to overcome, as my conscious and unconscious minds gave different signals on decisions made. Why is it that, contrary to my plan and strategy, I occasionally deviate from my plan through mixed feelings of fear, greed, vengeance, and overtrading?

One of the best pieces of information I learned was that trading with a conscious mind is only part of the picture. I had to deal with my psych surrounding trading.

I explored this further and found significant help from a professional, where I gained valuable insight into my psychology of trading. I enrolled in a program that would help me gain a mental edge in the trading markets. The program was led by professional sports psychologist Crede Sheehy Kelly, who drew parallels between sports and trading performances. Learning and practicing her strategies taught me a lot about trading and helped me deal with my personal trading challenges. Practicing what I learned from her also helped me create beneficial habits.

Now, I am closer to comfortably getting involved in future markets, practicing confidently, getting into the habit, and engaging myself in structured actions to achieve success.

A quotation by David Mc Nally is still displayed on the wall in my daughter's bedroom: "Your willingness to create a new dream or vision for your life is a statement of belief in your potential." This little sentence, taken into depth, gives such a positive outlook on life. It can be applied to any area of a person's dream or vision, which is a start in pursuing the potential that we all have.

This story is one of the many stories in my life, and I chose to share this experience because the journey seems unique regarding trading being overlooked by the public. It is notable also because males mainly dominate the trading industry. And I, as a woman, learned not to be intimidated by this paradigm, courageously dived into it, and overcame challenges to realize my dream.

The learning process never ends. Learning passively through experiences and, or actively by making an effort takes time, energy, and perseverance. In the process, I realized that any venture should be looked at through various lenses. Believing in your dreams and creating a positive vision of your goals makes the journey effortless as you drive into the path and feel that your instincts are serving you.

My personality trait kicked in selectively to pursue something unknown to me then, yet focusing on my vision is like following a trail that keeps me moving forward.

Monetary gain through non-traditional ways has always interested me. Instead of a 9 to 5 workplace, I always liked the freedom to work in the timeframe of my choice. I have flexibility in the workplace location, whether in my home office or while visiting places away from home, utilizing my computer.

The mental challenge, active mind, and positive mood are essential to trading. It had a hold on me and seemed to dominate effortlessly in time, and with this aura, it positively impacted my daily life.

In a nutshell, mainly the general public, not knowing the features involving trading, will generally label trading boring, as I was fixated on, thinking the same in my way at the beginning of my journey. First, mechanics is the central dominance in trading, involving numbers, statistics, possibilities, analysis, etc. However, the journey trains and disciplines your mind and thoughts intrinsically. It now has a positive impact on me.

What I learned is taking risks and yet knowing when to stop—having more patience and discipline to stick to strategies: market analysis and understanding of technical indicators, chart patterns, and market trends for executing trades.

I have been positively impacted in many other ways through this journey and the process.

Whatever age we are, there is always time to start something new. Like having better emotional control through the emotional highs and lows. Being more adaptable and flexible to stay ahead of the game. Managing time, plus focus and dedication. But more importantly, I want to be proud of myself as I learn and grow.

Although retired, besides my daily activities, I now have a new interest that excites me. You, too, can start something new, something you dreamed of - something you only dreamed of but never allowed yourself to do.

I am a Futures trader. My curiosity, love of mental challenge, and persistence led me to tap into this arena to gain monetary success and a sense of freedom to trade when and where I want. With these, I can impact the lives of loved ones and others, especially women!

This journey is to be continued – stay tuned for my upcoming book!

Now... back to my futures!

Manoushag (May) Emirzian

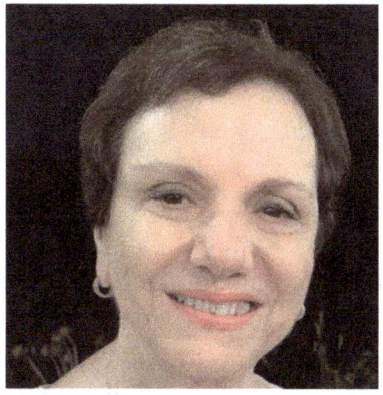

Manoushag Emirzian was born in Beirut, Lebanon, as the eldest of five children to Anna Stepanian and Garabed Beurklian. Her grandparents, survivors of the Armenian Genocide, hailed from Ainteb, Digranagerd, and Marash.

She attended Shalian Tatikian Armenian Evangelical School in Marash, Lebanon, graduating high school in 1971. Afterward, she worked as a secretary at an Armenian school for two years. Following her marriage to Krikor Emirzian, the couple briefly moved to Cyprus but returned to Lebanon due to political unrest.

Having previously obtained U.S. citizenship, Manoushag relocated to Glendale, California, where she pursued accounting at a business college. Upon graduating, she began her career with the Carpenters Joint Apprentices and Training Committee Fund (JATC), managing apprenticeship programs in trades such as construction and electrical work.

Her passion for connecting with people led her into real estate, where she helped families achieve homeownership. She earned her broker's license in 1994. Later, her curiosity expanded into trading, which she pursued alongside her other interests.

Manoushag has a deep appreciation for old classic films, historical sites, and the sciences—particularly health, natural sciences, and astronomy. Now retired, she enjoys day trading, writing, and engaging in life's simple pleasures. Her journey reflects a life defined by resilience, learning, and exploration.

A Life Full of Chances, Choices, and Changes

Armina Gharpetian

What's in a Name?

My name is Armina (on my legal documents), but my family and friends call me Armine (Արմինե). I often switch between the two, depending on the setting, whether it's a social gathering or a business meeting. "Armine" is a common name in Armenian culture, meaning "Armenian woman." But, until recently, I didn't know that "Armina" had another meaning in a different language. In German, it means "soldier" or "warrior maiden." In Latin, it signifies "noble" or "of high degree." And now, knowing the strength and grace carried by my name, I understand that anyone with this name could feel empowered to conquer anything they set their heart on.

A Journey Begins

"You're having twins! Did you know that?" These words, spoken by the nurse to my mother, were a complete shock. My parents hadn't known they were expecting two babies — a surprise that set the stage for an extraordinary life ahead. Born in the late 60s in Tehran, Iran, to Armenian parents, I was raised with strong Christian values and a deep connection to my heritage. My family, like many others, had faced challenges growing up in rural villages before moving to the capital city. Despite their limited formal education, my parents instilled in us the importance of knowledge, resilience, and the pursuit of a better life.

My parents taught us that no matter where you start, with faith, determination, and a clear vision, you can achieve greatness. Even without formal schooling, they worked tirelessly to ensure that all four of their children would attend college and reach for the stars. Their unwavering belief in our potential laid the foundation for the journey we would all take.

The Road Less Traveled

When I was just 10 years old, my world shifted. The fall of the Shah, the Iranian revolution, and the long years of war between Iran and Iraq brought uncertainty and hardship. Yet, through it all, I witnessed my parents' unshakable strength. Our family survived airstrikes and blackouts, and although I didn't fully grasp the gravity of the situation at the time, those experiences forged in me an inner resilience I would lean on later in life.

In the mid-80s, we left Iran, seeking freedom and opportunity in America. We resettled in Glendale, California, where my older siblings had already built their lives. It was here that I learned the true meaning of the American dream. Although we faced challenges — especially the language barrier — we held fast to the belief that anything was possible in this land of opportunity.

Overcoming Barriers

My first job in America was at a Halloween costume store, where I found myself interviewed by a local newspaper. As a shy teenager with limited English, I was hesitant at first, but that small act of stepping out of my comfort zone marked the beginning of my transformation. It wasn't just about selling costumes; it was about finding my voice. That article, now 34 years old, stands as a reminder of how far I've come and how important it is to take risks, even when you're unsure of what lies ahead.

Within three years, my twin sister and I graduated from Glendale Community College with honors. And to our amazement, we were both accepted into UCLA, a place we had dreamed about from our days in Iran. That moment, standing side by side and seeing our names on the acceptance list, was the culmination of years of hard work, faith, and belief in a better future.

Love, Family, and Purpose

Like many young girls, I dreamed of love, but nothing could have prepared me for the way it arrived. I met my husband unexpectedly, and when I say "love at first sight," I mean it. The connection was instant. It wasn't a fairy tale; it was real, raw, and perfect in its imperfection. That serendipitous encounter led to a beautiful, enduring partnership, and in May of 2024, we celebrated 30 years of marriage. Our love has grown stronger with each passing year, and together, we have created a family that fills my heart with joy.

Through every high and low, we've stood by each other. And, together, we've shown our three daughters the power of love, resilience, and the importance of following your heart. Our family is a testament to what happens when you stay true to your values and keep striving for the life you deserve.

Chasing Dreams, Even When They Change

I had always dreamed of becoming a pediatrician or family physician, but life had different plans. I developed a fear of dentists, particularly needles and drills, but instead of letting this fear define me, I chose to face it head-on. I decided to pursue dentistry — not only to help others but to conquer my own phobia.

It was a long road, but with the support of my husband and my unwavering determination, I earned my Doctor of Dental Surgery degree. What I learned through this journey is invaluable:

challenges are not roadblocks; they are stepping stones that push us closer to our dreams. You have to believe that every setback is simply an opportunity to learn, grow, and evolve.

Creating Balance, Making Impact

The next chapter of my life included becoming a mother, starting a dental practice, and finding a balance between family and career. With the support of my husband, I was able to create a life that was not only professionally fulfilling but also deeply personal. I later sold my practice and found my true passion in cosmetic dentistry, specializing in Invisalign treatments. It was a new chapter, but it never strayed from my mission: to serve others and to be present for my family.

In 2012, I decided to run for a seat on the Glendale Unified School District Board of Education. It was an endeavor that challenged me in ways I had never imagined. Public speaking terrified me, but I knew that if I was going to be a voice for the community, I had to overcome that fear. With the help of my campaign team and the unwavering support of my family, I was elected to the Board. I served for 9 years, always putting the needs of the students first.

Even after losing my re-election bid by a narrow margin, I was undeterred. I learned that sometimes the path we expect is not the one we walk, but that doesn't mean our journey is over. It's only just begun.

A New Beginning: Embracing Your True Calling

Now, at 55, I'm living proof that dreams don't have an expiration date. I'm an adjunct faculty member at Pasadena City College, helping to shape the next generation of dental professionals. I continue to run my Invisalign practice, and I find joy in the simple moments — like riding my electric bike through the city, cherishing time with my husband and daughters, and reflecting on the life I've built.

I've learned that dreams can evolve. They can shift and change, but as long as you're true to yourself and follow your core values, you will always find your way. Your story is your own, and only you can write it.

The Power of Following Your Heart

So, I challenge you — look at your own life. What is it that sparks your soul? What dream, no matter how impossible it seems, would you pursue if you knew you couldn't fail? What pattern have you followed, and where will it lead you next?

Believe in yourself. Believe in the journey. When you have a set of non-negotiable values and a clear vision for your life, nothing can stand in your way. Your dreams are waiting for you to take the first step. And I promise you, every step you take will lead you closer to the life you've always imagined.

You, me, all of us — we deserve a beautiful, meaningful life. Let's go out there and make it happen.

Dr. Armina Gharpetian, DDS

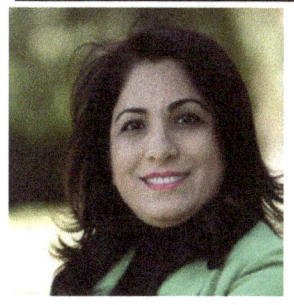

Dr. Armina Gharpetian was born and raised in Iran and migrated to the United States in 1988. She earned her bachelor's degree in Biology from UCLA and later obtained a Doctorate in Dental Surgery (DDS) from the University of the Pacific School of Dentistry in San Francisco.

Dr. Gharpetian has been practicing dentistry for over 25 years and owns a successful Invisalign office in Glendale, California. She also serves as adjunct faculty in the dental hygiene program at Pasadena City College and is an active member of the American Dental Association, California Dental Association, San Fernando Valley Dental Society, and Armenian American Medical Society. n 1994, Armina married her soul mate, Vartan Gharpetian, former Mayor of Glendale. They are proud parents of three daughters—Nazeli, Nayra, and Nelin. Armina is deeply committed to her community and has served on the Glendale Unified School District Board of Education for nine years, making a significant impact on youth and students in need. Additionally, she has held leadership positions in the PTSA for over two decades. Armina is passionate about giving back and serves on the boards of several non-profits, including the Glendale Youth Alliance, Glendale YMCA, Verdugo Hills Council Boy Scouts of America, Glendale Clean & Beautiful, and HealWithin International. Her dedication to community service and excellence has earned her numerous recognitions, including the Business Life *Women Achievers Award*, D&M Educational Foundation's *Woman of the Year*, Western Diocese of the Armenian Church's *Honoree of the Year*, Glendale Council PTSA's *Golden Oak Award*. Proud of her Armenian heritage, Armina treasures her culture and traditions while balancing her roles as a professional, community leader, and devoted wife and mother.

Website: https://www.invisiblebraces4u.com/
Facebook: https://www.facebook.com/armine.gharpetian
LinkedIn: https://www.linkedin.com/in/dr-armina-gharpetian-dds-1a35a523

The Resilience of Love
Jennifer L. Horspool

Have you ever wondered how strong women who seemingly have it all together find themselves in toxic relationships they can't seem to leave?

I do because I am one.

As I fell from the top of my game—revered within my company and among friends, colleagues, acquaintances, and strangers—to the depths of hell, I lost myself, my voice, my power, and my sanity. I struggled to climb back out. As I did, I discovered the *"No shit?!?!! Shit, you need to know."*

Here's what I learned.

Psychology says, "The trauma that happens to you as a child is the reason you have issues as an adult."

As I examined my childhood and compared it to friends who lived through literal hell, from abuse to molestation, alcoholism, and neglect, I thought, "I didn't have any trauma as a child, so what's my problem? Why can't I find love?" It seemed my life was always glorious until I fell in love, then it became a nightmare. *Why did this keep happening?*

As I started climbing out of the hell of my last relationship, I sought answers everywhere. At one event, someone said, "It's NOT the trauma that happens to you as a child; it's just, 'What happened in your childhood? And how did your brain record it?'"

Wait, what? Wow! That statement changed my life.

I never realized my issues could stem from something so seemingly benign, yet it's what has kept me from love my entire life.

I'm talking about the moments as a child when you learned messaging like, "You're not good enough," "You don't belong," "You're not lovable," "You're bad," "You mess up everything," or whatever your personal negative programming is.

When I started examining my childhood, I thought I had no serious trauma. I mean, sure, my parents divorced when I was 7 – but so did nearly everyone else's. And sure, my older brother turned into a jerk, so I turned into a momma bear to protect my little brothers, but overall, I came from a good family. We had great relationships and a good life. I knew I was loved. I didn't think I had childhood trauma. But when I re-examined—without judgment—unraveling my memories little by little, "What happened?" "How did it make me feel?" "Who was there?" "What happened next?" I discovered the situation that told me I was "less than."

I was 5 years old. And once it happened, it was never fixed, so I carried those feelings of abandonment and rejection throughout my life – collecting more data from each event that proved the theory true until I was hurting so badly inside that I didn't trust anyone to love me properly… only, I never knew it.

I remember the tears of that 5-year-old little girl and the sadness she felt when her three best friends, all boys, suddenly ousted her after discovering "Girls have cooties."

Yep. That's my big trauma. I mean, laugh as you must because, on the surface, it's funny. It's cute. Boys will be boys. But to me, at age 5, those words ripped my world apart.

Suddenly, everything I touched had to be sprayed with cootie spray. No one else's. Just mine. I was the only girl in this group. And before the cootie discovery, we were equals… then suddenly, we weren't.

Suddenly, no one wanted to play with the girl. They tried to push me in dog poo. These boys that I loved with my whole heart were rejecting me over a lie!

But life went on; the neighbor boys moved away, and we never played together again.

My family life

I was born to a family of all boys: four brothers and four boy cousins. No one wanted to play Barbie® like I did. I learned to play the boy way. We roughhoused, built forts, rode bikes, made human launch pads, and somehow, never broke any bones—oh, and we played sports.

We had the perfect street with a natural baseball diamond and football field. Those were our sports. And my insecurities were triggered in full force. I was such a girl. And no one wanted to hit like a girl, run like a girl, throw like a girl. I don't know why they never taught me, but I know I always felt like girls were less than boys. Boys were better at everything, and girls were pests – except for Tom Girls, which, of course, I was not.

That's what I heard throughout my childhood. And no one thought too much about it because that was just boys being boys. I was told, "Words don't matter. Ignore them. Go find someone else to play with." Not knowing I was learning avoidance patterns so, I could ignore the tears that flowed inside of me from the pain of rejection from the boys I loved – just go find fun elsewhere. So I did. And I pretty much did that my whole life – running away and changing the situation every time I didn't like how it felt.

Even after I got married.

I had no skills in fixing a marriage. I thought, "You're happy in your marriage, and you stay; you're unhappy, and you leave." That was all I knew. In fact, I was 15 before I figured out my parents' divorce probably was not caused by my dad forgetting to cut the watermelon before we left for the picnic that day.

But that was the day they started fighting.

Then Dad moved out, solidifying my new hidden perspective, "Men love you, and they leave you. You're the thing, then you're not. Get your lovin' in early because it's going to end."

I never knew this was my programming. I never knew I was the reason for my own pain and rejection in love. I discovered this in my late 40s. I had no idea that I viewed intimacy as dangerous, but I remember feeling the knots in my stomach whenever something didn't seem right.

As I look back at my dating history, I can see I like the fun ones. Nearly every one of them was an alcoholic who loved the ladies. I thought I was secure because I knew they were never going to cheat on me... until they did. And when they did – or even when they gave the attention I was craving from them to someone else – it felt like an explosion of pain would go off inside of me as I realized, "Oh no... it's true!!! I'm NOT good enough for them to remain faithful to." It was like a huge infection had been festering inside of me from years of pain pushed down into the depths of my soul, rotting with hurt... until one little prick (pun intended) opened it up and puss oozed everywhere.

I am not proud to say that I am the crazy girl – on more than one occasion. And I always felt justified. They were bad, I was good. They disrespected me and our relationship. They proved they didn't care. So to me, I felt like I had the right to be mad, hurt, angry, and psychotic. I felt indignant and justified. I did a lot of finger-pointing.

As I unraveled the memories of my life, I started to see how my beliefs formed; beliefs I never knew I had but that have been the basis for my decision-making throughout my life. I learned how my interpretation of events, words, and types of people, registered in my brain as dangerous or benign.

A riddle: If someone bumps into you, spilling your coffee, why did the coffee spill?

The easy answer is, "Because the person bumped into me, duh!?!" But that's not the answer. The answer is because coffee was in your cup. If you had been drinking tea, tea would have spilled. If you had been drinking water, water would have spilled. If your cup were empty, nothing would have spilled.

Same with emotions. Emotions are feedback. They tell us what to pay attention to and how to react: fight or flight, friend or foe, or freeze. Freeze happens in overwhelm. We call it stuck. But just because we're feeling an emotion doesn't mean our emotions are right or are even serving us well.

Someone brilliantly stated (and others repeated), "You will continue to suffer if you have an emotional reaction to everything that is said to you or about you. True power is sitting back and observing things with logic. True power is restraint. If words control you, anyone can control you. Instead, breathe and allow things to pass."

It's easy to feel emotions and say, "I'm feeling like this because THAT PERSON did THIS to ME!" We all feel like a victim sometimes. What I'm saying is there's more to it.

If you're feeling pain, guilt, shame, regret, depression, sadness, overanalyzing, or dwelling on events or conversations, you're living in the past.

If you're feeling anxious, worried, overthinking, asking "What if?" or imagining worst-case scenarios, you're projecting fear into the future and drawing negative energy towards you.

The reason you want to explore and heal is so you can live peacefully in the present, and no one can rock you. When you're living in the present, you get to experience joy, gratitude, empathy, clarity, acceptance, and peace.

Where trauma comes from

There is no accident, the family you were born into or the traumas you've experienced. It's by design for you to heal.

We're born with emotional intelligence from our ancestors for the world we're about to be born into. When that intelligence is triggered in our youth, it sets the path for confirmation that our emotional intelligence is correct. We're actually searching for it without knowing, and our souls recognize it as soon as it presents itself because we're wired to watch for this danger. This programming becomes our problem to solve. To study it, look at your life from ages 0 to 7, with age 5 as the sweet spot. That's when our brains are putting together the puzzle pieces of the world, discovering how it works and our place in it.

It turns out I come from a long line of divorced women who have a right to believe, "Men love you, and they leave you. You're the thing, then you're not. Get your lovin' in early, 'cuz it's gonna end." It goes back five generations… and that's only as far as I know.

So now, I look at my role in my family as the healer. I'm breaking the chain so future women in my family can soak up the love. So far, I'm successful. My one biological niece is the only grandchild on both sides of her family and the darling of everyone's eye. That doesn't mean she won't have her own issues to solve. She's likely got some other trauma we don't know about yet. We all get our share. We're supposed to. We can either look at it as it happened *to us* (victim) or *for us* (victor).

When you choose victor, you become empowered. When you choose victim, you're stuck. Most choose victim until we're enlightened to become our own victors. But you gotta give up the hurt feelings. You gotta forgive – not just others for their roles in your life, but also yourself.

Forgiveness is weird because it feels like you're letting the person off the hook when you feel they deserve punishment. Still, explore forgiveness. It's an important virtue.

Building Resilience

Today, I often think I'm healed, only to fall again. I finally decided to look at healing like hunger. No matter how much I heal today, some other unaddressed pain will rear its ugly head. I call it *The Artichoke Theory.*

In healing, people often talk about peeling back layers of the onion, but then all you get is more onion. And onions stink and make you cry.

I've rephrased it to "Peeling back the artichoke." Artichokes are delicious, but you have to work for them. They have thicker, tougher leaves on the outside and get more tender and fragile as you peel each layer until you get to the really fragile leaves hiding the icky, prickly guck. You must remove that guck to get to the delicious tender heart. That's healing. Rejoice in the deliciousness. And realize you'll likely be hungry again soon, and that's OK. It's normal. Peel another artichoke.

Healing is a practice. It's not about controlling your emotions; it's about diffusing them. You do that by understanding where they came from, what triggers them, and what role they play in your life.

Getting to know yourself means exploring your emotions and digging deep to find out what's making you feel that way. What's behind the feeling? Where did it come from? Why do you need protection? Is that protection still serving you? Are you ready to let it go so you can be free from its hold? When you're free, emotions are not driving your decisions. You can calmly make decisions to elevate your life.

Wrongs are not going to end. Bad will happen. But how you deal with it can change. The point is to build resilience so you can live in peace, where others cannot control you, and you can control your life journey even better.

Henry Ford's famous quote, "Whether you think you can or you think you can't, you're right," is relevant in every area of life, including love and emotional intelligence. If you're set on hurting, you'll hurt. If you're hurting and you don't want to anymore, explore.

Emotions are like computer programs in your brain. They formed for your protection. When you heal, protection is no longer needed.

Today, when I'm feeling wronged, it doesn't mean *they* didn't do something wrong; it's just that now I know their actions and behaviors are theirs, driven by their emotional needs, and my actions and behaviors are mine, driven by my emotional needs.

When I'm feeling good about myself, others cannot rock me, no matter what they say or do. I don't take anything personally. I let them be them, and I choose whether I want to share time with them or if I need a break.

We all have hurt. We all fail. We all doubt ourselves. Apparently, even Elvis wondered, "Will they still love me when they find out I'm human?" (*Loving Elvis*)

We all have the opportunity to change our lives each day… even when it feels like we don't.

Hostility, negativity, resentment, anger, revenge are all choices. Optimism, kindness, compassion, empathy, and forgiveness are too. How we live our lives is a choice.

So the next time you find yourself pointing fingers at others, notice how three more are pointing back at you. Find empowerment here. When you're empowered, you become the victor. Your energy elevates.

Energy begets energy. When you're hurting, you attract more hurt. When you're happy, you attract more happiness.

When you consistently give without receiving or receive without giving, when you push people away, when you act hurtful, when you erupt easily, it's not that you weren't wronged; it's that this viewpoint makes you a victim, and being a victim hurts.

Sometimes, there's comfort in hurt. Embrace it. Tell your inner child you're sorry for what happened to them. Embrace that child. Feel the love and forgiveness, then let the pain go. Release it so you're not stuck in the past, no matter how bad it was—even if you have to peel dozens of artichokes to heal it. When you can remove the emotional charges attached to these memories, that's when you know you're healed. That's resilience. Resilience is peace. Peace is love.

Jennifer Horspool

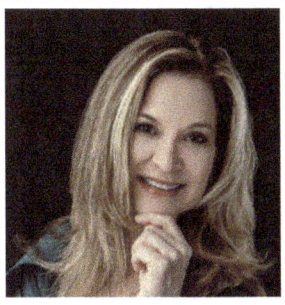

Jennifer Horspool is an international speaker, author, entrepreneur, and founder of Engagement PR and Marketing. With decades of experience, she has built and revitalized brands for companies ranging from Fortune 100 giants to start-ups, including Amgen, McKesson Corporation, Deloitte, Pepsi, Xerox, and the American Cancer Society, among many others. Jennifer's expertise extends across PR, marketing, messaging, and media, helping businesses grow from vision to multi-million-dollar enterprises and transforming brands into industry leaders. As a sought-after speaker, Jennifer has shared stages with A-list celebrities such as Mark Wahlberg, Gene Simmons, Christy Brinkley, Brooke Shields, John Travolta, Jillian Michaels, Dr. Phil, Jason Alexander, and prominent business leaders such as Steve Wozniak, Kimora Lee, Jay Abraham, Hugh Hilton, JT Foxx, Bill Walsh, Les Brown, Manny Lopez, and Moira Forbes, to name a few.

Her dynamic presence and actionable insights have earned her recognition as a leading voice in business growth and empowerment. A graduate of California State University, Fullerton, Jennifer holds expertise in Communications, Public Relations, Business, and Health Sciences. She is also an International Coaching Federation™ Accredited Business Coach.

When not working or learning, Jennifer enjoys time outdoors in parks, mountains, or beaches with her beloved dog, Bruno. A Corgi-Australian Cattle Dog mix, Bruno was rescued after weeks of sleeping under a friend's truck and has since become Jennifer's greatest joy.

Website: https://engagementpr.com/
Facebook: https://www.facebook.com/jennifer.horspool
Instagram: https://www.instagram.com/becomethegotoexpert/
LinkedIn: https://www.linkedin.com/in/jenniferlhorspool

Stitched in Fate

Zarik Kazanchian

I'm sitting here going down memory lane...I always knew I wanted to be a fashion designer.

My grandmother was a couture designer back in her homeland of Lebanon. I was born in Armenian, and as a 3-year-old girl, I would sit, watch, and marvel at how she'd seen - it was so fascinating how she would create an entire wardrobe with her tiny, delicate hands. While most of my cousins and neighborhood kids played outside, I would rather sit with my grandmother in her sewing room and sew clothes for my dolls.

To this day, I have kept memories, pictures, and certain ornaments that remind me of her, which means the world to me.

Blinded by the black dot.

Hello, my name is Zarik, and I want to shed light on how love, grace, and courage have been such an essential part of my life. Before things are cut, there must be a vision and a pattern.

It's 1995, and I'm living out my dreams. I graduated from the Fashion Institute of Design & Merchandising in Los Angeles two years ago. Now, at 22, I am an assistant designer, juggling work and being a happy newlywed, 7 months pregnant with my first child. Everything I've ever dreamt of is lined up and waiting for me - excited to see what is in store and where life takes me next.

On this day, I wake up... it's supposed to be just like any other day.

My daily routine consisted of putting on a fashion-forward outfit, kissing my husband goodbye after a lovely breakfast, and we each drove to our work. Except, this day did not turn out to be like any ordinary day. On this day, as I come to full awareness and open my eyes, I notice a large floating black spot in my left eye, as if it is blocking my vision. I think, "That's weird," I blink several times, hoping the spot will disappear. It's still there. What in the world - What's this? No matter how many times I blinked, it did not go away.

I remember rubbing my eyes and washing my face, sure it was just a particle that could be washed away. So, I rewashed my face and cleansed my eyes... but when I opened my eyes again, it was still there—freaking out a bit, thinking, what on earth is this, and where did it come from?

What am I to do about this?

Panicking, I called my husband from the other room while dialing my doctor. She listens and, with a calm voice, tells me to see my optometrist and have him get in touch with her- in the meanwhile, relax.

Relax? How? My husband and I got in the car and rushed to my optometrist's office just down the road from where we lived.

As we raced to the front desk, feeling more panicky because the spot was still there, I told the receptionist I needed to see the doctor urgently. I tell her that there is this unusual black spot from the moment I opened my eyes and that my vision is distorted. This has never happened. Sensing my distress, the receptionist calls the doctor. He walks in, greets us, and invites us to the exam room to assess what is happening.

After running a few tests with all the fancy optical machinery and looking into my eye, he explains what may be happening that I can't quite grasp. My mind is running in a million directions, and I can't concentrate on the information coming from his mouth.

Finally, as if hearing my husband's voice, I regain enough composure to focus and hear him say, "I've never seen anything like this throughout my career." That's it – I am doomed. My heart sinks.

What is going on with me? He continues to inform us of his findings and recommends seeing a group of ophthalmology specialists to diagnose better what is happening to me. As we left his office, the receptionist gave the information to one of the specialists. She requests that I make an appointment to be seen as soon as possible – this is an urgent matter. We make the appointment for later that same day.

Driving home, my husband does his best to be encouraging and talks me through this moment of doubt and panic. He reminds me not to freak out until we know what is happening. I face him and feel tears roll down my eyes – my seeing eyes. My heart is still racing. I can see the pain in his eyes, although he is trying so hard to be strong for me. I knew we were both scared and unsure of what to expect next.

At 1:30 in the afternoon, we walked through the doors of the specialist's office. By now, I could hardly see through my left eye. We met with the first specialist, and he started running different sorts of tests with what seemed complicated equipment. Leaving us in the exam room, he steps out to check and get the results of his findings.

After what felt like hours to me, he finally returned. He wants me to see another specialist before he can give a more qualified answer and recommendation. We go to another specialist's office the following day and perform the same routine. Fill out this paperwork, tell me exactly what happened, more tests with other fancy machines, and an even longer wait for an answer.

As the doctor walks into the exam room this time, I feel a chill. I can tell from his uneasy expression that this is not 'good news .' He starts his lengthy speech by saying that in the medical world, many diagnoses and problems are precisely what the textbooks say. And, of course, on the flip side, there are those rare cases that most doctors won't encounter during their practice only due to their uniqueness. However, mine is one of those rare, unique cases.

He continued to share that he needed to involve a few more specialists in his team to interpret the data correctly. The reason for his delay was to let us know he had to contact other specialists and ensure that they came to the best possible resolution and how to proceed next. My test results showed that I was born with a rare case of macular degeneration. I find this news shocking because I haven't had any severe eye issues in my entire life. Secondly, I'm only 22 years old! And thirdly, what is macular degeneration?

The moment of realization

He kindly and thoroughly educated us. This is "macular degeneration". It is an eye disease that destroys central vision, which explains the black spot. He shares that individuals with this disease have trouble reading and writing because of the visual obstruction they experience. What he shared next was astounding... he says this disease commonly affects individuals over the age of 60 – but I am not anywhere near half this age.

I need some clarification. So why is this happening to me? Why now?

What caused this? I am hyperventilating; I want to know why.

Feeling anxiety setting in and my voice trembling yet getting louder, I tell the doctor: "I'm pregnant" I am in the third trimester of my pregnancy." I hear myself speak even louder...I need to be able to see. I'm going to be a mom soon! What can you do to make this right? I can't have something like this happening to me. Not now.

The specialist shared that it is very possible that the stress of my pregnancy caused a hemorrhage in my eye, resulting in a black spot. I look at him, puzzled. Hemorrhage? But when? I didn't see any bloodiness in my eyes. I felt no discomfort until then.

It feels like I'm in a movie. He further explains that the test results are conclusive, with a hemorrhage in my eye that triggered a disruption in my vision. Then...I am in a daze. I watch his lips move, yet I do not hear him anymore. Just like the black dot...I feel myself in a dark hole.

Next, my husband is directing me out of the office. He tells him to make sure I go home and rest and to expect a call the next day with a game plan. I received a call the next day. I was told that my life would be different and that I must make certain adjustments. Due to my pregnancy and for the safety of my baby, all treatments will have to happen after the delivery of my baby and discontinuation of breastfeeding.

It's June 1995, and I just delivered my baby girl. She's not only beautiful but healthy in every which way. Crying with joy, I am relieved, especially after all the doubt, worry, and stress of what I have been experiencing in the last few months. Our family is whole, and our home is filled with much love and joy.

Months later, I scheduled my next appointment with the specialist.

Through the following weeks, I undergo more tests, only to determine when and what kind of procedure to do to stop the bleeding and hemorrhage from the back of my eye. After all that, they finally have something.

At the end of our appointment, the doctor informed me that for safety reasons, it was too late to perform any treatment, and surgery was out. The scar tissues have spread too far, and nothing more can be done to help my vision come back to normal. A good amount of my left-eye vision is lost, and I must learn to live with it for the rest of my life.

He asks if he can be frank and transparent with us. He shares that, in his expert opinion, I may become blind by age 40. To live my life to the fullest and accept my fate with the remaining vision I have left – and try seeing the brighter side of life!

In 1995, Western medicine and alternative healing had not advanced enough to find a cure or even an alternative treatment for individuals with macular degeneration.

Sitting in our backyard with coffee in my hand one afternoon, I lifted my head towards the sky and gently closed both eyes... basking in the sun, I listened to the birds chirping away. I listened to the beat of my heart. I heard the neighbor's dog bark, and for just a split second, I thought the life I envisioned, building, and looking forward to was turning darker. It was as if life was being snatched beneath my feet, and everything I worked for would be lost. Now what? I got nothing but...then I started praying a prayer my grandma taught me.

I asked the Lord to lead me to the right path, no matter where that is. I am to retire from the fashion industry and work alongside my husband, helping him grow and expand his dry-cleaning business.

Fashion is my foundation – designing is my Gift!

Fast forward 21 years; now it's 2017, and I am 44.

The good news is that I still have my vision! Although my left eye requires stronger lenses, I CAN SEE!

Deep down inside, I knew all is possible with the love of family and the Grace of God. I chose not to accept my fate, as indicated by the doctors. I decided to design a better life.

In October 2017, my husband surprised me with keys to my new bridal and tuxedo boutique. He gets extra brownie points for the best Gift ever! Today, I am the happiest and proudest owner and designer of KIRAZ Bridal & Tux in Glendale, CA. Although my journey started with many obstacles, I never lost faith that my dreams would return to find me. I AM and will continue to design, create, and fit more beautiful brides in their dream dresses!

Finding the light behind the darkness, the tread between the needle, and the trail that sways on the floor behind the bride's dress...is a testament to knowing I am exactly where I am to be.

Life is Grand.

Zarik Kazanchian

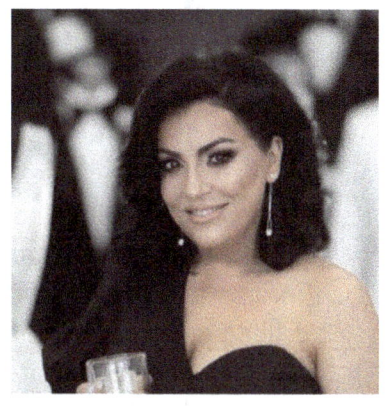

Zarik Kazanchian Born in Yerevan, Armenia, Zarik Kazanchian was destined to be in fashion. Growing up in the design world, she flourished as she started her ventures. From the age of three, she was taught how to sew by her grandmother. With many designers in her family, Zarik knew this was also in her blood. As an immigrant to America, she understood that she had to work twice as hard to prove herself. Her talents were advanced as she graduated from the Fashion Institute of Design & Merchandising (FIDM) in 1993.

Her career started as an assistant designer in Los Angeles, CA. She quickly dived into work and spent hours helping create an entire wardrobe collection. After an early retirement from fashion due to health concerns, she took on the position of Product Developer in 2007. Her new role allowed her to examine and critique artwork before it was finalized and sent to production. Some of Zarik's artwork has been turned into products such as keychains, magnets, and bottle openers. Collaborating with companies such as Hard Rock Cafe, House of Blues, Oakley, and Disney was a part of her daily routine. This experience allowed her to travel the world, understand the aesthetics of various cultures, and bring that knowledge back home to push new global trends.

Today, Zarik is a stylist who can be found in her boutique, KIRAZ Bridal & Tux, located in the heart of Glendale, CA. As it had always been her dream to be back in fashion, she broke barriers along the way and made this dream a reality. Styling men with various styles of tuxedos and suits and women in bridal and evening wear, this boutique has it all. "A second home," as Zarik would say, KIRAZ Bridal & Tux offers the attire and hospitality Zarik is known for. Inspired by her experience in fashion and product development, KIRAZ Bridal & Tux is the culmination of her talents. Facebook: @kirazbridalandtux/ Instagram: @kiraz_bridalandtux

The Power of Love
THE #FREEBRITNEY MOVEMENT AND ME
Lisa MacCarley

During what should have been a lazy, lovely vacation on the tropical island nation of Antiqua and Barbuda, an unfamiliar and powerful energy coursed through my soul, ignited my mind, and changed the trajectory of my life. As a tourist, I stood at a historical site, a former slave plantation called Betty's Hope, and I felt a sadness pass through me like nothing I had ever felt before. I stood there and wept; uncontrollable sobbing took over me. This sad and alarming moment was the beginning of knowing, too. For example, I knew I had to drop weight because I would be on television. I knew that for certainty, although I didn't know why, when, or any other details. I returned from that moment knowing something big was on the horizon.

That moment, which occurred during the week starting April 15, 2019, inspired me to practice being brave, too. I begin to swim beyond the resort's buoys to practice being afraid. I know it sounds odd, but I needed to build up my courage as if it was a muscle. I swam further away from the safety of the powder white sand each day and swam back, sometimes exhausted. I wasn't exactly afraid of drowning, but I knew there was a risk in being so far away from the safety of human glances. One night, I sang karaoke, which was more ridiculous than brave, but I wanted, in a strange way, to be laughed at and, maybe, humiliated. I needed this "practice" to solidify my belief that I would be just fine no matter what was done *to me*. Discomfort and even embarrassment was always temporary. Keep practicing being afraid, my inner voice said, so you can remember how brave you are.

The Britney Movement

That week, I spoke to "the Universe" – the great unknown and mysterious – and promised to do something to stop the torturous dysfunction of the California probate courts that had haunted most of my professional life. I knew that policies and procedures put in place by overworked, untrained, and unsupervised judges were wreaking havoc on families through a combination of incompetence, cronyism, and misogyny. I knew that the judge's reliance on epically stupid "reports" by utterly untrained, unsupervised, and unaccountable lawyers was the problem, and I said so, aloud, on a cell phone video I still have.

Unbeknownst to me, another member of the legal community was also making a life-altering recording that very same week. A paralegal from a law firm involved with the Conservatorship of Britney Jean Spears left a message for "Britney's Gram." The shocking claim from the anonymous caller was that Britney had been placed in a mental health facility against her will.

This call would ignite the small group of Britney's fans who had begun to hold rallies against the conservatorship. For them, there was something more urgent about freeing Britney, and they loved her that much. The conservatorship seemed more suspicious and sinister than ever to them. I had no idea.

I have often wondered about timing since I learned about this strange synchronicity: was it just a coincidence or a call to a greater destiny?

Upon my return to Los Angeles, I eagerly aligned with other probate court activists and found no shortage of "probate court" victims. Armed with irrefutable evidence of incompetence and cronyism, I met with California senators and assembly members. I even walked the halls of the Capitol in Sacramento to speak with legislative aids. I gathered up my newfound courage and flew twice to Sacramento to speak to the top tier of the California judicial community for three whole minutes at a time. Voice quivering with fear, I addressed the inconvenienced faces of the California Supreme Court and their peers. At the same time, I tried to explain the "trauma, exploitation, and abuse" being experienced by probate court litigants in Los Angeles County. They could not care less. This is all recorded, too.

I was unstoppable for the balance of 2019 and the first two months of 2020. I found allies. I challenged judges and threw shade at the report-writing "court-appointed" liars, I mean, lawyers. I felt invincible, and frankly, it was a blast to push the buttons of the white, old, retired men who made up the vast percentage of "court-appointed" what-have-you's in Southern California. Leave it to the patriarchy to make up policies and procedures that undermine justice. But what could they say? That I was wrong? I wasn't. That I was unprofessional? Less professional than writing gibberish and submitting it as a "report?"

That was the craziest thing: I was speaking truth to power and knew a more powerful force was protecting me.

In every sense of the word, I went to a full-court press to make sure that what had been done to the families of two elderly, incapacitated Bettys, Judge Betty Lou Lamoreaux and dear Betty Roberts, would never happen again. Not to my family or yours. Never again. I created Betty's Hope, a charity to protect people from the broken system that inflicted trauma, exploitation, and abuse. I was fueled by the hope that things could improve, and I could see it. Feel it. Practically touch it.

And then, in an instant, everything stopped. March 15, 2020. A life-threatening pandemic had reached us, killing us, scaring us, scarring us.

- COVID19.
- The murder of George Floyd.
- The civil unrest.
- Racial inequality.
- Earth is Dying.
- Stay home. Be home.
- Stay safe. Be alone.
- Offices closed.

The optimism I had experienced, genuinely believing that we, the activists, were on the precipice of real change, vanished, and I was left in a deep, dark depression. I had let go of hope for reform, change, or even acknowledgment that things could improve.

There was simply no point to life after all. Based on what I watched on the evening news, Evil was winning. I knew I would never leave my children to wonder why they weren't worth living for, but I was calculating how much longer I needed to be on this planet. I was planning my escape. Not just the general concept but the actual details. Where? When? How? The "why" was the easiest part. Letting go of hope was the worst thing anyone could experience, and I had ultimately let go.

Breaking the sad, dull existence of pandemic life came a call from a young man I never heard of: Kevin Wu. Kevin had gotten my number from a colleague who had heard about my pre-pandemic activities and asked if I would meet him at a #FreeBritney rally. To be honest, I had no interest in that at all. While we, those involved with the Los Angeles County probate courts, all knew "the legend" of Britney Spears' conservatorship, the judge and the lawyers involved disgusted me. Honestly, I wanted no part of it or them.

But Kevin persisted. Oh, what the hell. Leaving my house that morning, I remember telling my daughter, Ali, that I didn't want to go, but I had made a promise, so I was stuck.

As an attorney, I am used to going places I don't want to go, literally and figuratively. That is part of the job. So, off I went to fulfill a promise.

I Am Visible

Feeling invisible, wishing I was invisible, I recorded another moment of embarrassment, my prescience scarier still. I was handed a bright pink megaphone and released years of frustration: I complained about the judges doing what they were told to do by court-appointed counsel who wrote these stupid reports. Oh, how I hate those silly reports written to sell out "justice" for only $250 an hour. And the judges love the reports, no matter how ineptly produced and misleading.

Was I scared? Standing in front of the courthouse, screaming through a fuchsia megaphone, calling out to my colleagues and the judges for the disastrous system they had put in place? You better believe it. But, at that moment, I had nothing to lose.

After my not-so-brilliant rant, the two women of Britney's Gram, Tess Barker and Babs Gray, approached me and asked if it was confirmed that I was a conservatorship attorney. They asked if I would review some of the documents, they had located concerning how Britney's conservatorship was started. Of course, I said. It was the summer of 2020, and there was nothing else to do, so we began exchanging emails. At first, I thought this was naughty, looking at documents placed under a protective order.

Honestly, I wish I could say I saw the whole picture right away, but I did see that something was wrong right off the bat. Attorney Adam Streisand (yes, a relative of Barbra's, but don't ask me how I still don't care...) had shown up at a hearing, at Britney's request, and was not allowed to represent her. That was a clear violation of the law. Hurray for me, I had been an attorney for over 25 years, and this much I knew: Britney was irrefutable, undeniably entitled to an attorney of her own choice, no matter what anyone else had to say, including Dr. Spar. That's Due Process, Constitutional Law 101.

This is the point where I knew that the young people of the #FreeBritney movement were right, and their claims were righteous. No aspect of the conservatorship could be excused or legitimatized once Britney was denied the attorney of her choice. But wait, there was more: Jamie's attorneys, the judicial officer, Reva Goetz, and the court-appointed favorite, Samuel D. Ingham, III, all agreed that Britney would never be given the documents filed to deprive her of life, liberty, and property. They conspired to violate Britney Jean Spears' constitutional rights from one side of the courthouse to the other.

The #FreeBritney movement was now, in the eyes of the law and the media, 100% legitimate and not a conspiracy theory or whatever they tried to label it. The love and commitment of the #FreeBritney movement had unraveled an evil conspiracy, but no one from the political side was still concerned.

As it turned out, New York Times' Samantha Stark and Liz Day, however, were watching, listening, and recording. In February 2021, they released a brilliant documentary called "*Framing Britney Spears.*" If you haven't seen it, put down this book and watch it. Pay attention, most of all, to Adam Streisand's interview. That moment when he excuses his dismal representation of Ms. Spears with "You Don't Know What You Don't Know" pains me every time I watch the documentary. I want to shake him and shout, "The Law, Adam, you didn't know the inalienable right of every single person facing the loss of life, liberty, and property." How the hell can you show up in a courtroom and not know the basics: the constitutionally enshrined right to counsel of your own choice?

The following week, Netflix came out with its version of "What Happened to Britney" in the dark comedy *I Care A Lot*. Dianne Wiest flawlessly depicted a sort of elderly woman who was placed in guardianship without notice, without a medical declaration, and without competent counsel to defend her. Just like Britney Jean Spears. (Again, coincidence?)

In my pandemic quarantine, with a pair of fluffy cats as my trusty companions, I kept thinking, oh, for sure, someone must pay attention to this. They were. Federal and state legislators were interested in having their names associated with freeing Britney. Politicians and journalists, at long last, became interested in "fixing" the nation's probate and equity courts. (They still haven't, but change is challenging.)

The #FreeBritney movement became internationally recognized for its intuitive, virtuous, and pitch-perfect advocacy. This was no longer about Britney's fandom concocting rumors; this was about the LBGTQ+ community getting loud and proud and shouting it from the rooftops. How could anyone not be in awe of this Power? This Love?

Jamie Spears and his lawyers, including Sam Ingham, who had been paid $10,000 a week since mid-2008 to represent "Britney's interests," were busy negotiating, trying to keep the conservatorship in place, but with changes.

The #FreeBritney movement was stronger each day and more persuasive by the minute.

On June 21, 2021, Britney Spears spoke to Judge Brenda Penny, which was stupefying. Britney completely vindicated the

#FreeBritney movement and more. She explained how unheard she felt that she wasn't aware that she had the right to an attorney of her own choice, that she didn't know she could petition to terminate the conservatorship without being evaluated. She revealed that she had been lied to, scammed, defrauded, and violated in immeasurable ways by a phalanx of fools and quasi-criminals who enriched themselves greatly at her expense.

Alas, Judge Brenda Penny did what she always does: nothing. She thanked Britney and didn't change a thing. She could have fired Sam Ingham. She didn't. She could have ordered that Britney be provided with all the documentation that she had been deprived of over the last awful and unlawful thirteen years. She didn't. She could have told the truth and apologized for participating in the scam. Again, she didn't.

But this was, absolutely, the beginning of the end of the conservatorship. A few weeks after Britney's public statement to the Court, the court-appointed counsel resigned, and Jamie's phalanx of lawyers must have recognized that the "fee for all" was over. A petition to terminate the conservatorship was filed by Jamie Spears and set for hearing on November 12, 2021.

My Mission

Over Labor Day weekend in 2021, I began to piece together another "great mystery" of Britney Spear's conservatorship. Mr. Streisand affirmed over and over again that Retired Judge Reva Goetz had told him that she had a report from gerontologist Dr. James Edward Spar, informing her that Britney lacked the capacity to retain him (even though she did retain him), and that was why he left the courtroom, taking any semblance of justice for Britney with him.

I carefully went over everything about the first weekend Jamie was appointed as Britney's temporary conservator, and there is one thing I can say with certainty now. There was never a Dr. Spar report in Reva Goetz's hands. The entire conservatorship was based on a hoax, a lie, a scam, and a sham, and great effort was made to cover that all up for over thirteen years.

From a foundation of pure love, the #FreeBritney movement emerged as a force that inspired a groundbreaking documentary and catalyzed legal change, leaving an indelible mark on the world. In reflecting on my role, I believe I became a conduit of that profound love, experiencing a sad yet otherworldly energy during the pivotal week of April 15, 2019. Love became my catalyst, empowering me to find the courage to speak out, even gracing the television screen as I discovered the Powerful She within. This journey serves as a testament to the transformative power of love, urging all women to harness their inner strength and stand united in the fight for truth and noble causes.

Lisa MacCarley

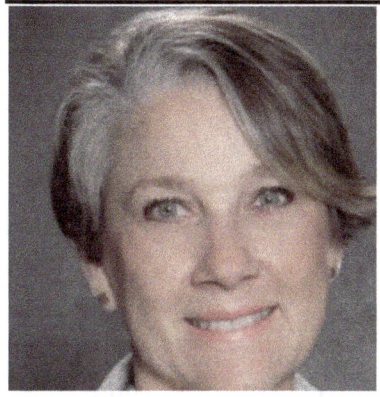

Lisa MacCarley has been a probate and conservatorship attorney since 1993. She became a reform activist in 2019 when she realized that the probate court inflicted needless harm on consumers. In 2020, she learned about Britney Spears' constitutional rights violations and became internationally recognized as a leader of the probate court reform movement.

Lisa attended Loyola Law School and was admitted to practice law in California in 1993. A former New York state resident, she attended the State University of New York College (SUNY), Cortland.

After visiting Los Angeles to thaw out after four long years in the arctic tundra of upstate New York, Lisa fell in love with the City of Angels and has lived here ever since. Lisa MacCarley worked as a law clerk in 1990, and by 1997, she had established her practice in Glendale as an estate and probate lawyer.

Facebook: https://www.facebook.com/Lisa-MacCarley-108930551578044
Instagram: https://www.instagram.com/lisamaccarley/
LinkedIn: https://www.linkedin.com/company/83068361

Wandering Wind
Sanaz Manouchehrian

Once upon a time, in the vastness of the universe, a spark of existence ignited, giving birth to the story of life. The formation of planets, including our own, set in motion an incredible journey.

But our story still needs to be completed. Today, as we stand at the precipice of possibility, our actions and choices shape the narrative that future generations will inherit. It is up to us to determine the path that the story of life will take. So, let us begin this chapter with reverence and a deep understanding of the interdependence of all living things. With empathy, knowledge, and a sense of shared responsibility, we can weave a tale filled with compassion, equality, and sustainability. The story of life is ours to tell, and the pen is in our hands.

I take a pen in my hand to write, but I face an empty mind as if it wasn't me who experienced all that pain and suffering. Yet it is because of those challenges that I became who I am today. I will do my best to write about this woman who once built her identity based on a story - telling it as if it's her reality. Now, more accessible than ever, she can boldly say, "I am more than a story."

One could perhaps say that life begins with a person's entry into the world or even earlier, and mine, for sure, is a tale of the struggle between death and life from the beginning. I wasn't meant to stay alive. In July of 1970, I was born prematurely and came into the most challenging time of my parents' marriage.

On the one hand, my physical body was under massive pressure to cope with the new environment, and on the other hand, my mum was having a hard time supporting me in terms of feeling safe and loved. Perhaps being resilient and eager to stay alive shaped me to endure the difficult times to come. I consider them my life force.

It took me a long time to learn that the early traumas of my life, and even those of my parents and ancestors (trans-generational trauma), had created an unconscious system of beliefs and patterns. This system made me feel unsafe and unfocused most of the time, and, as a result, I have always been indecisive and overwhelmed. Being placed in situations beyond our control, which we can consider as bad luck or an accident, plays a significant role in shaping our character and future. My childhood, schooling, career choices, marriage, and even migration were all influenced by a set of circumstances out of my control - for example, the Iranian revolution, war, etc.

The closed and suffocating atmosphere of those years, the limitations and cultural pressures in society, bitter memories of my father's arrest due to his political activities, and the unwarranted harassment my family endured by the morality police would make me think of escaping Iran.

All these events, outside pressures, and internal turmoil eventually turned me into someone who knew only what she didn't want. I did not want to suffer. In those days, nobody spoke of trauma; nobody thought that we all suffered from distress, depression, and anxiety. Nobody knew anything about the massacre of lost hopes in our society, and like my other friends, I concealed all my desires behind closed doors.

To escape the constant pain and turmoil, I chose to marry at the age of 24 to my ex-husband, a 25-year-old decent young man studying abroad. We married within two weeks of meeting – not knowing much about each other. He chose me, and I remained passive and silent.

So, things had happened to me, not by me.

After we married, we left Iran to go live in the Netherlands. From the first day, I was not happy with my marriage nor with immigration. I couldn't find a place where I felt a sense of peace and comfort at home. The world outside was unsafe and emotionally cold; inside, it was unsecured and frozen. To survive this emptiness, I had to be more flexible yet forget my wishes and needs. This flexibility made me let go of a part of who I was, my desires, and my boundaries. Gradually, I adapted to everything. We moved from one home to another, from one city to another, and even to different countries like wandering wind. Each time we changed location, a piece of me was left behind. I did not allow myself the chance to fully connect with people, the new place, the community, or the environment.

For 12 years, we fought, argued, and clashed repeatedly. Each of us was busy with our work and studies. But when together, we'd be engaged in quarrels - merely surviving life until we decided to have children. My motherly instinct made me think I was ready to share my love. We had stable incomes, secure jobs, and a sense of stability. Yet, we didn't know how to love each other, most importantly, ourselves. Two years later, I got pregnant with my son and again two years later with my daughter. My life became busy caring for the children and him earning money and providing for them. The gap between us grew even more.

One day, as I was filling out a form to apply for a passport, I noticed that there were only three options for us to choose for marital status: single, married, or widow. My mind and soul were searching for a fourth option. The option I was looking for could reflect my feelings of being abandoned, lonely, and confused within my marriage. I did not fill out the form as the voice in my head kept getting louder and screaming, "You're left out."

I walked out of there feeling more confused and overwhelmed. I knew I had to do something in this situation about my behavior, pattern, and even co-dependency. I had to give in or to change.

In the summer of 2010, with my two children and just two suitcases, I headed to Malta - a small island south of Italy to start a new and better life.

During the first year, everything was new and exciting, even for my ex-husband; I hoped this change could bring a new dynamic to our relationship. I thought there was a better chance of saving my family's life on this beautiful island with warm and sunny weather. I even found a stable job in a pharmaceutical company. Life took yet another turn, and our marriage got worse with each passing day.

My circle of friends expanded, and I climbed higher in my career in management positions. All the while, our relationship became more complicated till I reached a point where, after three years of constant threats to lose my children, I decided to divorce. He packed and left for the UK. Once summer, my children wanted to visit their father for the summer holidays.

A few weeks later, while waiting for their return, I received a message that they won't come back. That moment was the day of true darkness and a new radical change – a WAKE-UP ALARM inside my being.

Rumi said, "Die before you die." I experienced death while I was alive. I always considered myself as an invincible building, with a solid foundation, but at that moment, an earthquake shattered me into the same dust. All my self-perceptions, the image I had built of myself and presented to the world, along with all the dreams and expectations associated with it, were buried in a grave within me.

I lost completely myself and felt like a failure. I left my job - the company's name and reputation were no longer associated with my identity. I was not married. I did not belong to anyone or anywhere. What was the meaning of my life?

The nervous breakdown.

My tears fell for no good reason in the following days and months. Whenever I saw a young boy or a girl of my children's age, I would start crying. Even seeing white or black cats, which they had one, would make me break down and feel terrible. I cut off all contact with everyone I associated with because of my cultural shame and embarrassment to share what was happening in my life, terrified of being judged.

I was constantly asking myself: "Why? What did I do wrong as a mother? Who am I now? Why did I marry this man? How did I choose him?"

I felt guilty one minute and righteous the next. I constantly judged myself harshly. I was a victim and had the scenario to prove it – but then, at another moment, I was innocent. I would write and rewrite all possible scenarios that would not have happened if I had done this or that. If I had said, acted, given, and the list went on and on. Or if I had made a different choice, they would still be with me.

The fact was that I felt miserable, not because they were not living with me but because I felt rejected and not wanted. I felt 'not good enough - not lovable'.

The situation brought all past behavior patterns and beliefs to the surface. A voice from within me was screaming, like a wandering wind that echoed in my ears. This voice seemed to originate from past pains and sorrows hidden in my heart – in my being. It appeared as if everything was entangled, and my emotional apparatus had become overwhelmed. The voice was dangling with unspoken whispers of my soul, and I was caught up in my thoughts. "Who Am I?"

During this period, life showed another side; I met a man who became my partner. Someone who loves me for who I am without any judgment. He once told me, "One day, you will come to see what I see in you now." During this time, I got acquainted with my dear mentor, Ursula Maria Bell in the field of spirituality and family constellation practice and, through social media, got in touch with Liza Boubari.

My journey to self-discovery had begun! I started paying more attention to my needs and listening carefully to the voice within. I was able to gently wrap my wounds and scars with love and got on the path of healing. Gradually, I collected all my broken pieces and embraced them. I put each piece back to its perspective place and honored myself as a whole.

Practicing mindfulness has helped me be more present and evident in my head and stick to asking the essential questions for every situation. Is this true? What would my feelings be if it were true? And if it is not!

And the best thing for me has been stepping out of the story and connecting to the reality of the now. The more I separated myself from the past patterns, the more I stepped out of my fears and into the new comfort zone. I chose to stop considering myself as a victim and nagging about my destiny as I realized that this was my path, my own unique path that belonged to me and only me. There is no right or wrong; it is all about experience and raising consciousness.

I started a new life with my loving partner. My children had limited contact with me – sometimes a short message when they needed something. For nearly five years, I longed and worried for my children. My savior and the only thing that helped me cope with my anxiety was a mantra that came to me in one of my meditation sessions. I have been repeating this mantra since.

My love will always protect them so they can have a healthy, happy life even if we are apart. With all my heart and soul, my children are connected to me with this invisible bond of love, so in due time, they will return, and we will live together. I have always believed that life does not wait for anyone. We live in the moment if we become more present and mindful, and this is the way we can show our gratitude for life– be more present.

This is why I took another chance to start a new life—enjoying life with my beloved partner and taking advantage of every opportunity to learn and grow. I participated in workshops and courses like Twelve Steps, NLP, CBT, Systemic Constellation, and family therapy. I grabbed the chance to learn about mystic Sufism and ancient Eastern philosophy to find the answers to my questions about my life.

I have pondered the roots of my sufferings. Where did this feeling of abandonment and inadequacy come from? It wasn't just mine; it started way before me. Perhaps from my mother, yet my grandmother had similar experiences. I may have inherited these attributes of confusion and disorientation from my family, community, and environment. Fear and anxiety, shame and guilt come from the society and the blaming culture in which I was raised. That culture had ingrained in me and many women like me the belief that we are less than others and that whenever something goes wrong, it is our fault.

Systemic constellation has helped me to get done with the past and to release my anger towards my parents and myself. I want to honor them for who they are with love and forgive myself for what I have done and have not done. This work helped me change my perception of the story of my life. I could let go of the old story and see it differently. Without the complex and challenging experiences I endured, I would not have been the person I am today. I am grateful to life for providing me with the lessons to learn.

Well, who am I without my story? I am a child of life, a child of the great force.

Who are you without your story? You are a child of life as well. In fact, I was never left out or abandoned by anyone; I was unable to remember my true self (re-member).

I can be a parent to my inner child and reassure her that those days are gone. Reality resides within the moment, and, most importantly, I am in the circle of self-love. Today, my children are grown up. They have become young man and woman with a bright future ahead of them. We spend quality time together, and our bond grows stronger each day.

I am now trained as a systemic practitioner and family constellation facilitator. I am a coach, holding seminars and training on self-development, organizing retreats, and helping women recognize their strong points and highlight their true potential. I help women who don't know how to overcome their inner fears or have a vision or mission for their life, who don't know how to say no, and who consider themselves a total failure when they fail in one project. Women who identify themselves with family, husband, and title. Women who are experiencing guilt and shame tend to hide their femininity and keep their beauty inside.

If you experience the same, I want you to know you are not alone. Your treasure hides in your discomfort. In chaos, you can find ways. Through suffering, you grow. You are not your story. The story helps you to connect with your true self. Use this tool to know yourself: your beliefs, patterns, your shadows, your strengths, and your gifts.

Now, take your pen - write your hero's journey and design your future.

Sanaz Manouchehrian

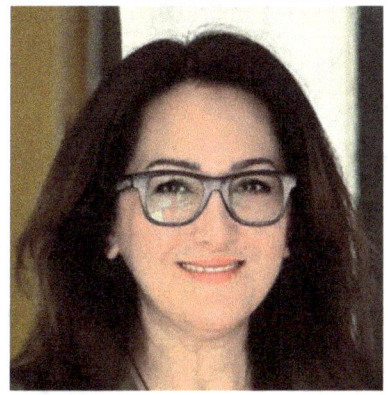

Sanaz Manouchehrian is a 53-year-old Iranian living with her partner in Malta and Germany. She first immigrated to Nederland in 1996, then moved to Belgium and the UK. She is the mother of two and works as a life coach and systemic constellation practitioner with a background in Molecular biology and Biotechnology from VUB University in Brussels.

Sanaz got her second degree in medical and pharmaceutical research. Meanwhile, she has been working with refugees as an interpreter and integration. After moving to Malta in 2010, she joined a pharmaceutical company, worked in an R&D and sales management position, and became interested in communication and neuroscience.

After experiencing a massive change in her personal life and burnout, she focused on a deeper search for healing and self-development. After several years of learning different principles and therapeutic methods and participating in many workshops and trainings, she found systemic constellation. She believes this to be the most fascinating and helpful method for dealing with transgenerational trauma and self-discovery.

She completed her training at an advanced level for family constellation and system intelligence. She is a coach for an educational charity organization helping children and teenagers in Iran. She works primarily with women who are mothers, coaching them to handle situations with their children to build healthier relationships. She is now involved with an international project with CI Academy for Constellation.

Facebook: https://www.facebook.com/Sanaz1970
Instagram: https://instagram.com/sanazm_1970

Against All Odds
THE JOURNEY OF TURNING MY MESS INTO MY MESSAGE
Alina Martin

Is all this a dream? Is it a nightmare? Or it's both. Intertwined together in a journey, I'm currently experiencing what we call life. You see, my story is different from anyone you know you'll ever meet. My story is different- then again, I'm unique!

My life didn't pan out how I wanted or hoped - but this is how it was meant to be. They say each of us has a destiny to fulfill. All of this is part of a greater purpose - my purpose: to share this as no one else can tell except for me and me alone. There is this saying, "Whatever happened, happened, and it couldn't have happened any other way."

I was born an only child to two Armenian immigrant parents, which, in and of itself, makes my story more unique. I was raised in a Christian household, and my faith in God has helped me through all these years. I was diagnosed with Cerebral Palsy at birth.

Cerebral palsy affects muscle control and movement. I have spastic Ataxic Cerebral Palsy. Spastic means "stiff," and Ataxic means "without order." There are times when I have no control over my movements. They happen involuntarily. I am still determining when they will occur. Further, I have jerky movements which I cannot regulate.

My story can't begin without bringing up my incredible family and the two homes that will forever be engraved in my heart and soul: my childhood townhouse where I was raised and my grandparents' house. Both homes hold the keys that unlock my past. You see, my life began within these two homes and the people in them—these houses built me and gave me a solid foundation. These walls have heard my silent cries from pain, joyous occasions, and laughter. These walls have witnessed my victories, tragedies, pain, and loss. Both homes gave me the pillars to one day stand on.

My Strength

I would not be who I am today or where I am if not for the unconditional love and support of my family-- my parents, to be precise. They are the best mom and dad God could have bestowed upon me. They have been through hell with me. Almost anyone with half a brain can understand that raising a child is not easy- never mind a stubborn girl with special needs.

My mom has been my most prominent advocate - whether in school, at home, or any place else. I recall my elementary school days when several teachers would want to force me into special education classes, and mom would stand her ground to keep me in general education- she knew and truly believed that I was more than capable.

She is why I survived the twelve years of school and graduated with Silver Honors from high school, and I just graduated from college with Gold Honors. Mom has given up so much in her life to care for me. For me, she is the Powerful She and personification of strength. Whether taking care of me, her mom, or going through her own challenges, mom is the pillar of our home and the true embodiment of a superwoman (without a cape). My father has worked twice as hard to be able to provide me with a good life. I would not be who I am without my parents and my family as a whole.

There have been a whole host of occasions throughout my life when I have asked myself, "Why me?" regarding my disability. As I write this, I came up with an answer to my question: to use writing as a medium to share my story and be a voice for the voiceless going through the same things I am. If my story can touch just one person, then I've accomplished my goal.

I now believe God created me like this because He knew He could use me to help others. Maybe He ordained me to tell. I've constantly been told that I have a writing talent. At times, I wonder if I would be passionate about writing if I didn't have speech impediments (due to my CP). Writing is a form of communication when I cannot express myself verbally or be understood by people.

2008-2009 was a miserable year where an emotional scar was engraved into my existence. That year was like a nightmare, except I was not asleep but wide awake and present. My fifth-grade teacher was honestly the worst human being I have ever been unfortunate enough to meet. She was a novice to the job with no prior teaching experience, let alone teaching special needs students. As the year progressed, I began struggling in my studies—notably in math. I failed all the math tests. When this happened, my teacher and the school decided to enroll me in RSP (Resource Specialist Program) classes. They would take me out of my classroom every day (where we learned new lessons) and relocate me to the RSP class, where the teachers there would have me work on assignments below my academic abilities. I had to take exams from which I was absent when the lesson was being taught.

Having cerebral palsy and being stuck in a wheelchair with spasms can be a challenging and complex experience. I have the exact needs, wants, and aspirations of a non-disabled person. My most significant want is to be included and not excluded from society. I want to feel included. While it is true that I do have my fair share of limitations, I'm also capable of doing many things. I have my unique ways that might not look like how an abled body person would do them.

It's essential to recognize that each person's experience with cerebral palsy is unique, and they may have their ways of coping, adapting, and thriving. Completing simple everyday tasks that no abled-bodied person thinks about comes as a challenge to me. Getting dressed, brushing my teeth, fixing my hair, eating, and talking are all struggles that I deal with that an average person doesn't have to worry about

All these struggles give me immense frustration that no one else can understand or relate to unless they experience it. This frustrates me, especially when people ask me why I do them. When I know that I'm not initiating these movements. However, When I'm relaxed, these movements subside drastically.

People with disabilities have feelings and want to be acknowledged just like anyone else. What I mean is that when you see a person in a wheelchair, don't make their disability your sole focus. You might be surprised how smart and well-rounded we can be. Often, in public, I cringe when I am stared at. It feels like I am being judged and put into a box because of my physical appearance.

My Advocate

A week before my IEP (Individual Education Plan), we had taken a math test, which the entire class had bombed- even her so-called best student. My then one-on-one oversaw the teacher transferring the class's score into the grade book. She noted that the whole class failed that specific test and that I was not the only one. She shared this with my mom. On the day of my IEP, this teacher dared to scold my mom for my below-average performance, saying that she believed RSP services would serve me better. So, my mom demanded that she cover the individual students' names and only reveal the scores that each student received. Distraught and visibly shaken, she refused to do so. My mom responded, "So this means the problem isn't my kid; it's the teacher."

Due to my speech impediments, the RSP grew determined to make me use assistive technologies to communicate in school. My mom and I were against this proposal, but the school insisted. Claiming it would make me "more independent."

Yes, I know I do have speech problems, but I am in no way non-verbal. Yet, I was forced to use a computer on which I'd type my thoughts, and it would say them out loud as if I were a zombie. My teacher encouraged me to participate in class discussions by using this device, which I despised doing. Every time I had to use it, I'd cry. As it turns out, the school insisted I use it because they profited from providing it. In my next IEP, my mom demanded they take that thing away from me, telling my teacher to encourage and motivate me to speak and participate in class.

Like that was not bad enough, the head of the RSP threatened my mother, saying if she were against me using assistive technology, she would take her to court. That's when my mom was forced to hire an advocate to speak to these lowlifes because they wouldn't listen to her. My mom was left with no other choice but to pay another person to say the same thing as she did, and these idiots listened to the advocate but not my mom. Unbelievable.

They say that good things can happen during a storm. This is true. When the school year began, I was with my aide, who had been with me since kindergarten. A year before, when I was in the fourth grade, my aide left on maternity leave, and I got assigned a new one-on-one. Remember I said I am stubborn and do not do well with change? It is hard for me to adapt to new and unfamiliar ways, not because I want to be hurtful. Unbeknownst to me, this change was one of the greatest blessings of my life.

When fourth grade ended, my mom chose a new aide, Mrs. Anoush, to assist me through middle school. Anoush was different from any of my previous aides; she has been like a second mom to me—she always believed in me and what I was capable of. She always pushed me to my limits, like my biological mother. I think she knew how to work with me because of her nephew, who had the same disability...This is a classic tale of how God will use your hurts, pains, and stories to heal somebody with a similar life story. The fifth grade was the year I discovered my love for writing lyrics.

The summer of 2010. This was the time that my beloved grandma, my dad's mom, passed away. We called her "Ma." I was only thirteen years old. This was the first loss I had experienced. Losing her is no doubt one of the hardest things I had to endure. I miss her every day. Gone, but never forgotten. I carry her with me wherever I go.

My Courage

2015 - Because of my love for television, I realized I'm interested in writing for TV. Watching TV dramas and sitcoms, I wonder, "How do writers develop these storylines? How are scripts written?" This sparked an interest in me, and screenwriting was something I could pursue.

Years before, I had sent handwritten letters to big-time Hollywood entrepreneurs like Oprah Winfrey and Ellen DeGeneres, introducing myself and asking for a shot in the industry as a writer. I also sent a mass email to studios like CBS, NBC, E!, and Columbia Records. Two days later, I received a reply from NBC stating that they do not collaborate with outside influencers. Although disappointed, I was just beyond happy to have gotten a reply. Two days later, I received an email response from the Director of Multimedia at CBS. He said it is not in his purview to assist in matters like this, but he just wanted to say hello. But then, I got the email I was praying for.

I got an email from the then-manager of CBS's Entertainment Diversity and Inclusion department. She stated that colleagues within CBS had read my email, and her boss asked her to contact me. In her email, she commended me for having the guts to ask for what I wanted. She invited me to the CBS lot in Studio City for a meeting and a tour. My mom and I got an unbelievable tour of the CBS lot and a once-in-a-lifetime opportunity to visit the sets of CSI Cyber, Brooklyn Nine-Nine, The Insider, and Entertainment Tonight. My very first time on a TV show set was beyond imaginable. While on the set of E.T., we met and took pictures with Mr. Cameron Mathison and Mr. Kevin Frazier. We also got to meet the Co-Executive Producer of Undercover Boss. This may be my BEST accomplishment to date...I did it with my determination. Throughout the years, I have kept in touch with them.

My Journey

2016 - My proudest accomplishment was graduating high school. I remember wearing the red graduation cap and gown. I was so proud; my soul was filled with joy. I accomplished something significant and worthwhile. I felt the world was a blank slate, and my future was all in my hands. Listening to the commencement speech, I wrote the words.

Graduating high school was bittersweet. This school had been my second home for four years. Some of the best people I have ever met were at this school. When my name was called on stage, the audience gave me a standing ovation. I was recognized with silver honors to go with my diploma. What made that graduation extra special was that my family—my grandparents, aunts, cousins, and mom's uncle- flew in from Virginia just for me.

Post my high school graduation, I decided to take a gap year from school only to determine what college to attend. I set my sights on attending New York Film Academy to study screenwriting. Falling into my safety net, I enrolled in Glendale Community College.

2017 - Going to school then was a very different experience compared to post-Covid. Attending college was a huge adjustment. I did not have an aide, so my mom became my one-on-one. She attended all my classes, took notes for me, and wheeled me from class to class.

2020 - The pandemic hit, and life as we knew it was forever changed. Just like everyone else, I began taking remote Zoom courses from the comfort of my own home. I took two journalism courses. That resulted in me writing several newspaper and magazine articles published digitally and in print.

June 17, 2023, I graduated with Honors from GCC, earning my Associate of Arts degree in Mass Communications.

February 2023 – my one and only grandfather went to join "Ma" and his older brother in heaven. This was the second most significant loss of my life and perhaps the most tragic. The day he passed was no doubt the worst day of my life. My "dada" was a very instrumental figure in my life. He was like a second dad to me all my life.

He was there for me through my best and worst of times. He played a significant role in my upbringing—we were always together in all that we did. In many ways, I am who I am today because of my parents and grandparents, especially Dada. He was funny, kind, loving, and most of all, a fighter- never afraid of anything, not even death.

His passing took a toll on me, yet I again found the strength to carry on. After all, he'd instilled in me the desire to forge ahead and not give up. To Dada --- I miss you each day and love you always and forever. Until we meet again- J'attendrai.

Alina Martin

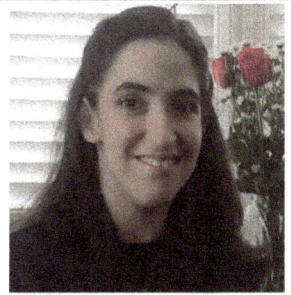

Alina Hope Martin is a 25-year-old writer, author, and lyricist. She will graduate from Glendale Community College in June of 2023 with Honors, earning her associate of Arts Degree and certification in Mass Communications. Alina was born and currently resides in Glendale, California.

She graduated from Glendale High School in 2016 with Silver Honors for maintaining a 3.8 GPA throughout her four years. She is passionate about writing, television, and music and wants a career in all three. Alina has Cerebral Palsy.

Her disability has presented her with a great deal of challenges but also with many opportunities that she wouldn't have otherwise had. Alina's family, friends, and, most importantly, her faith have made her who she is.

Alina is working on publishing her book of poetry later in 2023.

Alina would like to thank her aunt, Liza Boubari, for giving her a medium to tell her story. "Love you, Auntie!"

Facebook: https://www.facebook.com/profile.php?id=100009830563840
Instagram: https://www.instagram.com/aliina____martin/

Discovering The Powerful She in Me
Nancy Matthews

As I sat in my chair, attending yet another seminar to build my business, little did I know that the words about to come out of the speaker's mouth would change the trajectory of my life in every way. Spiritually, emotionally, and financially, shaping the very core of who I would become and discovering who I was always meant to be.

His words came in through my ears and bore deep into the pit of my stomach, creating a rousing stir so strong that I jumped up and out of my seat and shouted, *"Yes, that's me!"*

Shock and surprise flooded my mind as I wondered... "Who said that? Was that really me?"

I was quickly followed by other women jumping out of their chairs and rising to the call to action.

What were the words said that caused such a stir in me and other women in the room?

The seminar was called Monetize Now, led by Tony Martinez, to improve my public speaking skills so that I would better engage and inspire people to take action. As the event kicked off and Tony looked around the room, seeing only 20 women in a room of 100, he said: "Why are there only 20 women here? We need more women speakers. We need more women leaders."

Flashes flooded my mind of all the women I've seen struggle to make it up the corporate ladder. Very few women leaders and even fewer exhibited their authentic and powerful feminine nature as they sought to break the glass ceiling set in place by the good old boys' club.

That was my moment of being called to step into The Power of She, a power I didn't know existed, let alone a power that I possessed.

Tony engaged and inspired me to action that day. I am forever grateful to him for igniting the spark that led to the creation of the Women's Prosperity Network, which, through its formation and ongoing global community, continuously reminds me and reinforces The Powerful She.

What's so surprising about this is that I never even belonged to a women's group. If you had told me I would be leading a worldwide women's organization one day, I would have told you that you're looking into someone else's crystal ball. I was never one to have a circle of women friends; I mostly hung out with men and, in fact, never felt like I fit in with other women.

Through high school and college, I felt inferior to the popular girls - they were prettier than me, thinner than me, and more attractive than me. While I wasn't a Tom Boy, I wasn't a girly girl either and felt like the odd man out, so to speak.

When I jumped out of my seat, claiming my place as a woman leader, I first saw it as a leading woman real estate expert and speaker. To look at my life at the time, I had it all - two wonderful children, solid relationships with my sisters and several close friends, a beautiful home, a successful real estate business, and good health. What wasn't apparent was what I felt under the surface, like a duck sailing gently across a lake, with its feet paddling feverishly to stay above water. I was paddling feverishly to keep it all together, juggling the many demands of my time and attention while wondering if the struggle, overwhelm, and simmering discontent I was feeling was the price one must pay to achieve success.

I had followed all the rules (well, most of the rules), went to college, got decent grades, got a good job, and always sought to give my best.

How could the image of success I had been working towards bring me so little satisfaction, fulfillment, and happiness? Upon finding it, I had been chasing the holy grail, only to discover that my cup was empty.

I had followed my mother's model of being a strong, independent woman, providing for myself, and moving up the corporate ladder in a primarily male-dominated industry - the legal profession. I felt accomplished after escaping a path in my early 20s of drinking and drugging, an unexpected pregnancy, and choosing to have the baby and raise him on my own. I had successfully advanced from just getting by, living paycheck-to-paycheck, to owning my own home, having several real estate investments, and running my own business. I was driven by the desire to give my children (and myself) as much sampling of life's buffet through travel, sports, music, and art.

I worked hard and played hard - just like 'they' said to do, but it was becoming harder and harder to keep going. Something was missing, and I had no idea what it was. Little did I know then that all that "doing" kept me from being happier, more relaxed, and fulfilled.

Picking up the baton that day to be the leading female speaker and expert in real estate, I was invited to be part of a team of four women to create a new women's seminar company. Their vision and mission were to provide women with education, resources, and opportunities to be empowered wealthy women. The idea intrigued and inspired me, and I set about closing my real estate company to devote myself full-time to this new venture. I headed into it with gusto, doing market research, business planning, and hosting focus groups of women around the US. In the process, I learned so much about women and myself and found the missing piece I yearned for. A piece that was never missing but buried deep inside me under a mountain of false beliefs.

The Missing Piece: I am good enough. I'm better than good enough, and I'm more than enough. I am worthy just by my being, even without all the doing.

It was time for me to stop comparing myself to the popular girls - they also have unique worries, doubts, and fears.

It was time for me to stop believing I had to work hard to prove my worth; my birth determined my worth.

It was time for me to stop trying to climb to the top and rest as I uncovered the art of receiving and allowing.

Through mentoring, self-discovery, and reflection, I became aware that the success model I was following was based on discipline and determination as the driving forces. And while those are worthwhile qualities for achieving goals, they require an excessive amount of effort and lots and lots of doing. No wonder I was feeling exhausted and empty. There had to be a better way, and thankfully, there is!

The better way is found by having your BEING guide your DOING. This begins with pausing long enough from doing it to become aware of the energy within you that's running the show.

Let's take a look at the energy that was running my show. The qualities I relied upon to achieve success, discipline, and determination are masculine energies. Receiving and allowing are referred to as feminine energies, and I had little or none of that energy running the show. My masculine energy was full throttle most of the time, causing me to feel completely out of balance. I didn't know how to remain successful and slow down to allow and receive; quite frankly, I didn't even get what that meant. Then, I was invited to simply be the egg.

Nature shows us the qualities of masculine and feminine energy in the act of creation. Consider the sperm that moves forward with enthusiasm and determination to make it to the egg in a highly competitive environment while the egg simply waits, allows, and receives. She doesn't have to "DO" anything. Her role in creation is to BE for life to begin.

Creating our best life comes about through the dance of balancing being and doing, creating harmony between our masculine and feminine energies, and utilizing them appropriately to experience greater flow, ease, fulfillment, and happiness.

Before this, I knew that masculine and feminine energy differ (haven't we all heard of John Gray's *Men are from Mars and Women are from Venus?*), but I hadn't considered how these different energies were operating in my life.

As a single mother, I assumed the role of both mother and father, with the masculine energy of the provider and protector leading the way.

As a business owner, I assumed the role of boss, tapping into the model of the men I'd seen as hard-working, determined, and disciplined to succeed.

My feminine energy was reserved for nurturing my children, intimate relationships, family, and friends.

As I continued my journey of self-discovery and embraced the power of femininity, I realized that I had neglected an essential part of myself for far too long. The balance between masculine and feminine energy is crucial for overall well-being and success, and I was determined to find that equilibrium in my life.

To do so, I delved deeper into understanding the nature of masculine and feminine energy. The masculine energy embodies qualities like assertiveness, logic, and goal-oriented behavior, while the feminine is associated with intuition, nurturing, and receptivity. I began to see that both these energies were present within me, just waiting to be harnessed and harmonized.

As a business owner, I had been solely focused on the traditional male model of hard work and discipline to succeed. But now I understand that I could integrate feminine energy into business practices. This meant embracing intuition, collaboration, and creativity to find more effective and fulfilling ways to achieve my goals. I now rely upon my intuition, my being, to guide my doing and not only have greater peace and happiness - but I've also experienced more tremendous success!

(If you'd like to harness the power of your intuition, visit NancyMatthews.com/Intuition for free training, where I share the methods for deepening your connection to your intuition.)

The transformation was not easy and still requires attention and intention. It took time and conscious effort to undo the conditioning that had led me to prioritize the masculine aspects of myself while suppressing the feminine ones. However, with each step, I felt a growing sense of wholeness, peace, ease, and fulfillment.

Embracing my feminine side also meant embracing vulnerability and authenticity. I learned that my strength lies in my vulnerability (thank you, Burge Smith-Lyons). It has allowed me to connect more deeply with others, and as I embraced authenticity, I found that people resonated more with my genuine self. It's the secret to fitting in as you stand out as the powerful, divine being you were created to be.

By nurturing my feminine energy, I began to find joy in the journey rather than merely chasing the pot of gold at the end of the rainbow. Life has become a dance with all aspects of myself, where I can be ambitious and driven while allowing myself to savor the moments of rest and rejuvenation. I learned to appreciate receptivity's power, be open to new possibilities, and enable the universe to work its magic. And I've found the magic is the best part!

As I continued to explore and embrace my feminine energy, I realized that this was not just a personal journey but a calling to support other women to do the same. Women's Prosperity Network became a platform for women from all walks of life to come together, share their stories, and support each other in embracing their authentic selves. It's a place for women to be honest, get real, and achieve accurate results!

Looking back, I can't help but marvel at the journey I have been on. From feeling like an outsider to leading a global movement, my life has been transformed by the power of embracing my femininity. I have learned that true empowerment lies in embracing all aspects of ourselves.

As we continue to progress, let us always remember the transformative power that lies within us.

Together, let's continue shattering the glass ceilings, rewriting the narratives, and creating a world where everyone is free to embrace their authentic self and soar to new heights.

So, to all the women out there, Embrace Your Powerful She, for within it lies the key to unlocking your true potential and changing the world. And to everyone, remember that true empowerment knows no bounds, and when we come together, we can achieve the extraordinary.

As you sit in your chair today, may you find a spark to ignite and awaken another part of you that has been lying dormant, stepping into the next level of expression as your extraordinary, vibrant, and authentic self.

We may not have it all together, but together, we have it all!

Nancy Matthews

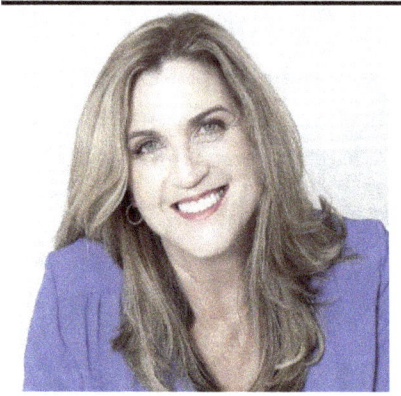

Nancy Matthews is a Leadership, Sales, and Marketing Expert known as The One Philosopher & The Visionary with Guts. Her unique blend of creativity, business savvy, and exceptional understanding of human behavior causes audiences to sing her praises far and wide.

She is a six-time best-selling author. Nancy is a sought-after international speaker and global leader. She has shared the stage with today's top business and thought leaders and has been regularly featured throughout the media.

As a single mother of two (now all grown up), Nancy knows first-hand how to juggle the many demands of our time and energy to achieve extraordinary results. She founded The People Skills Academy and Women's Prosperity Network. She works with growth-minded individuals who want to increase productivity, results, and relationships (life and business).

She's a music lover and a long-time fan of Bruce Springsteen and The E Street Band, having seen over 80 of their shows. One of her visions is to use the power of music to spread The One Philosophy, and she's co-written a song with Fiz Anthony, "Everyone's The One," that she plans to sing with Bruce Springsteen one day!

Website: https://nancymatthews.com/
Facebook: https://www.facebook.com/NancyMatthewsSpeaker/
Instagram: https://www.instagram.com/nancymatthewsspeaker/
LinkedIn: https://www.linkedin.com/in/speakernancymatthews/

Single Flower in a Concrete Street
Gia Razando

Have you ever figured out how a single flower can bloom in the middle of a concrete street? Where are its roots from, and how deep do they go? Who planted the seed? Who nurtured it? How did it know it could survive? Does it have a plan on how to survive? Does it have feelings? After all, it is alive. Does it rebloom after it dies, or do you have hope that it even might? Does it know it will one day be picked from the cracks it grew from, just to be admired only to become an inspiration for others!?

Hello! Let's dive into the woman that represents this flower. Come along as I share a sneak peek of my story; after all, it doesn't entirely matter how much I feel alone because there are chances that many others feel like how I do. Perhaps the very things you, too, feel SO alone with is for you to know you are never alone. There are billions of people in this world with similar pain that we choose to deny or express.

Let's start towards the end, as I am extremely dyslexic and have lived my life backward, upside down, crossed over, down low, up high, and somewhere in the middle of time...

Breathing heavily, my chest pounding, nerves throbbing. What is he going to say to me?

I stand in front of an entire room of my mentors and peers. I'm just waiting to be harshly criticized. I can handle anything with my imaginary sword as I am the Goddess and THE Warrior. I needed this to be able to stand in front of strangers. I quiet my thoughts. My palms sweat, but I keep my arms down to my side and my chest wide open. I welcome the feedback because I control what I do with it. He tells me, "Gia, You are the billboard for what is Possible in a world of transformation. Your war has ended; you can put your sword and armor down. You have fought to become who you are, and now it's time to enjoy the woman you have become and the life you have created to be the leader you were meant to be. You live from a place of possibility and resilience".

I was ready to fight back, but instead, I stood there. I could hear myself breathe intensely. I knew I had entered a place where I would be the reason to help others, not be held back. From this 6-month intensive training program, I will become a trained inspirational/motivational facilitator. Since I built my media company, I have offered different ways to experience forms of healing through photo sessions with me. I also became a life coach and stayed involved in programs that allowed me to reach out to the masses and be an interruptive impactor in people's lives.

Let's talk about being responsible for breaking down the concrete attached to your feet. The barriers surrounding your heart. The mechanisms you have chosen to numb away from the aches and pains of enduring. Everything you've built from survival has served a purpose at some point. Then come the stories you tell yourself as a form of justification as to why it's okay to have the patterns you have and the armor you've carried. We all have built a relationship with this survival kit and might even find more comfort in knowing how tough we are because of our ability to be prepared to fight any fight that comes our way.

Today, I can share the story of a child that was repeatedly raped, lived in shelters and on the street, traveled from school to school, was bullied for my race by all kids, and was left to fend for my mom and brother in countless ways. The unbelievable story of relentless love to the only fighting I do now is to get people to wake up from their pain and see they, too, can be much more than the stories of pain they have survived.

Do you tend to hide behind your mask? Hiding behind the stories you tell? What if you were to create a life where you inspired people? Can you imagine a world where the pain that you and I experienced through life didn't determine how we made decisions? But to create a present that involved healing, love, and being an example of what's possible in forgiveness. Are you extra curious about me yet? Since I only have you for a chapter, let's jump into a glimpse of my life.

I ran to school every day to be safe from home.

At school, I was bullied, jumped, humiliated, written on, choked, kicked, and thrown against walls. White kids hated me for not being white enough. Brown and black kids hated me for being white or "lying" about being mixed (because of my features). They either used me to teach someone else a lesson or took their anger out on me.

And this was still my safe place because at home:

Are we looking for food here? There are so many smells and layers of dirt. Why do they get to shop in the store for food, but I've got to climb into this dumpster? Okay, Mom, I'll find something.

***

I need you to take this with you to school, Mom says to me. I need you to keep it safe because he will never think you have it. It's our only way to save so we can leave in the middle of the night.

***

"Peaches, Get into bed with us! Peaches, don't make me ask you again...Get into this bed! Peaches Marie, if you don't get into this

bed, I will make you miss school! Get into this bed! You will have me a child!!! Come make him happy. If you loved your momma, you would come to get into bed with us. He wants to snuggle you! I will shave your head if you don't get into this bed". They won't stop calling my name and listing what will happen if I don't come to them.

***

LOCK AND LOAD, she yells as my brother and I scramble to grab what will fit in our laps. We know those words mean move now, and don't ask questions. I know I'm in charge of loading the hatch with her stuff, and I get to have what fits in my arms. We drive for hours and sleep in the car. It's the safest we ever are, in our seat buckled-in, not being touched. My mom got the bruises, and I have memories of her laying on the floor staring into my eyes while I covered my brother's.

***

If you live in this house, you will be mine. The more you make me happy, the more I will not hurt your mom or brother. If you tell anyone about what happened here, your mom, brother, and you will have more hell to pay than any relief you will ever have. What happens at home stays at home.

***

"If I call you at school tomorrow, you will know I made it through the night, but If I don't, just know. I need you to tell the cops they can find my body in the pasture. I'm too tired to keep living this life. Someone will adopt you; you will be better without me. I don't want to live and can't be your momma anymore".

Imagine how I felt as this child. What would I say if I could use my voice without punishment?

Hello, I'm Peaches Marie (GIA). Sometimes, I'm also Sister, Dorchika, Love Child, Brittany, Giovanna, Roller Girl, Jenny Jones Girl, and other names I don't understand why they call me. I am dyslexic, and it's hard to memorize some things. I don't think the same as people my age or adults in my life do. I observe people and think about what they have experienced to make them feel like they do.

I love to sing, dance, and express love in any way I know how. I try to make people laugh and do everything possible to make everyone around me feel unique and loved. I'll give you my food, shoes, clothes, protection, and understanding. I want to feel like they are essential.

I have a mom who isn't whole. She has a mental illness and doesn't know how to protect her children. Instead, I have someone who wants a sister and best friend, who doesn't protect me but instead puts me in situations where people can easily hurt me, adding to the list of things I can't say.

Notice how my inner child doesn't sound like a child?

It's because she/I didn't know what a child looked or sounded like. She was her mom's best friend, sister, and Warrior: her brother's protector and everyone's hero. Cinderella would never meet her Fairy Godmother. She was the cut-up garments that hung from her body. The homeless child is on the corner of the gas station. The scraps and left behinds for everyone's rummaging.

She was, "Yes, ma'am, no, sir." She was surviving. She was a soul trying to make it out alive and protect and spread love to as many as possible while getting there.

What my inner child wasn't? She was NOT disrespectful, angry, mean, deceitful, weak, emotional, or entitled.

More than anything...she was never a child. She is ME!

When I survived my childhood and got away from the control of my teenage household, I knew how I wanted my life to change. I immediately started building an empire of amazing people to experience life with. I knew what I wanted to do with my life and wasted no time impacting people's lives from what I survived. I had a voice inside of me tell me often (at such a young age, it didn't make sense), "Your life is special; it is meant to endure so that you can support others," and would teach valuable lessons. Standing outside the crowd and being willing not to fit in might mean not being loved, but it would mean utilizing my stories and ways of thinking to get others to take ownership of their life. I want people to see that no matter how much the people in your life can penetrate your body/mind/soul, you still have a voice and choose to take ownership of who and how you become in this lifetime. I knew that every ounce of my time, energy, and love would be focused outward, supporting people to stand up after the current pulled them under.

We can live from anger, or we can live from a passion to create a new story.

During my adult life, when I thought my childhood traumas were not a part of my adulthood, I felt capable of anything. I had "done the work" to realize my strength and saw I didn't need to handle my traumas like most might. I thought I had become invincible because I had survived all that life had thrown at me... Until One day...

I was in the ocean and was surprised by a wave. It knocked me over, as the waves of life can sometimes do. This wave, however, was followed by another and another and then a hidden current, turning me upside down and sideways in the water. Whenever I found the sand to dig my toes in and pushed up to gasp in the air, another wave would hit and back under, and I would go. I was tumbling underwater, fighting for my life as my knees hit obstacles I couldn't see, and my hands and arms got cut up and scraped. I needed a hand or anything to grab onto for stabilization, but it was me with me out there. My muscles were weakening, and the chances to catch a breath had only happened a few times. I found myself with no energy left to fight. I closed my eyes and surrendered, thinking, "This is it." I survived all that to die in a way that no one even noticed I was dying.

I woke up on the sand, burning from the cuts and scrapes on my limbs, grateful for the rise and fall of my chest. I was surprised that the ocean hadn't taken me. No one saw this fight between me and the sea, this battle for life. No one saw my hand reaching out for a hero (yet again) that wasn't there (yet again). No one saw the will to live, leading me to surrender to the idea that I could save myself. No one saw me become my hero (time and time again). This moment, this fight to live, was me with me, except I was not a child anymore; I was an adult fighting to live. She is ME

I could allow my past to victimize me over and over.

I could live out my adult life feeling like I am owed something, given that I never should have had a chance to survive everything I did.

I could walk around blaming all men for the men in my life.

I could walk around with impenetrable armor around my heart.

I could be the most untrusting person you have ever met.

I doubt anyone's ability to look outside themselves to help someone else.

I could live only thinking about what I wanted and doing things that only made me happy.

I could blame and be bitter and unforgiving.

I could live with a victimized mentality and park on everyone's emotions.

I didn't have a hero, so why care to feel bad about anyone else struggling?

Given my past, I could stay angry because of situations that seem so easy to go through.

Instead, I choose the impact I want to have on this world:

To take ownership of what I do with the details I have experienced.

To show up time and time again for people.

To stand authentically expressive in a room of people who might think I'm too much.

To dance when no one else is.

To laugh as loud as it comes out without feeling bad for it.

To make eye contact and smile without a word needing to be said.

To hold the door for strangers and buy random people gas.

To acknowledge everyone no matter what they are doing/wearing/saying.

To notice the mask everyone puts on each day.

To stand up to get people to realize their past does not define them.

We can choose from a place of responsibility and ownership – and how we want to be.

So much energy is put towards holding onto pain. Pain that you have gotten so comfortable with having that you might find yourself having built a relationship with it. I invite you to look at your life and be willing to see all the ways you have allowed your stories and pain to become a part of your ID badge. To know you must mean to understand the struggles you've survived to reach where you are. But to BE is to create the person you want to be today. One that people find themselves proud to know and love. One that would be colorful and boundary-pushing. One that would need to rise repeatedly to be what is required in transformational opportunities.

The words BE THE CHANGE, make for a pretty quote on a magnet. But what if you lived your daily life challenging being victimized? Instead, choose to focus on all the ways you could give love, break down walls, and be what wasn't provided! Be what you might have once chosen the opposite of.

Just because You might have created an identity that once suited who you were doesn't mean that you can't intentionally choose to face yourself and the pain you might have created or endure and actively practice a daily choosing of whom you say you want to be and be so committed to this that you would stand in the fire for anyone or thing to breathe life into what you say you want and whom you want to be EVEN with the stories you might have to tell.

I know who I am, how I change with life experiences, and my daily energy level. I may not fit in any specific mold, and I understand that in a world of billions of souls, I might rock some boats and create discomfort in people. A little boat-rocking is a price I'm willing to pay if it means I, along with you, set our chains down and allow love to seep into our veins and fill those deepest crevices of our hearts so that we begin to heal.

To the victims and the victimizers (because you never know who is carrying shame for something), what if today is your day of becoming your own hero? Choose to grow through all the walls you've created. Set down your chains and have more energy to love and be loved.

With Love – GIA

Gia Razando

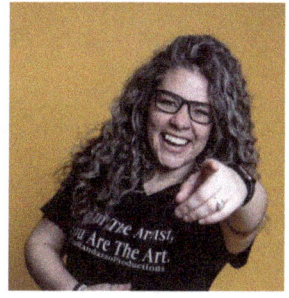

Gia Randazzo is a renowned international fine art photographer and a trained Ontological Facilitator. She focuses on the physiological reframing of internal dialogue to help others be fully present and accepting of their mental, physical, and emotional bodies.

With specialized training and over 20 years of experience, Gia goes far beyond the traditional photo session to create a sacred space to access full transparency in a healing and transforming way.

Gia is a chameleon who can give support in many ways. She utilizes her skill set for fine art portraiture, motivational public speaking, and creating and facilitating retreats, workshops, and group healing experiences. She has photographed many high-profile clients in over 15 countries, offering the exclusive opportunity to bring her studio to any client in any location, regardless of where they are. With a warm, vivacious manner and magnetic personality, Gia draws others in and uses her life experiences and training to instill positive concepts within others. The chapter within is only a short glimpse into an extraordinarily colorful life.

Website: www.GiaRandazzo.com
Facebook: https://www.facebook.com/GiaRandazzoProductions/ and https://www.facebook.com/giarandazzo
Instagram: https://www.instagram.com/gia_randazzo

Overcoming Obstacles and Peaks
Natalie Regg

I did it. As the realization of what I had just accomplished hit me, I couldn't keep the silly grin off my face. I kept reliving the past 21 days and the events that had brought me here. The Nepalese I passed on my descent greeted me with knowing smiles as I pressed my palms together and said, "Namaste." They knew the route I had just traveled.

The Annapurna Circuit in Nepal has been voted the best long-distance trek in the world, consisting of 145 miles through beautiful scenery and local villages. The path reaches its highest point at Thorung La Pass at 17,769 feet. The definition of a "trek" is a long, arduous journey, especially one made on foot. In hindsight, that definition was spot on. My trek began with three flights: first from Los Angeles to Guangzhou in China, then from China to New Delhi in India, and finally from India to Kathmandu, Nepal. I had hopped on each of those flights with nothing more than my backpack full of gear and two traveling companions who were sisters and family friends.

I picked up the pace a little as the excitement flowed through me. The phrase "You did it" kept repeating in my mind. I had pushed through many challenging days these last three weeks, including spraining my ankle and hiking through it and the type of mind games that come with exhaustion and long hours of isolation. I was so proud of myself.

During the easier sections of the trek, I reflected on why I was in Nepal and what I was doing next. I was in the middle of a divorce. It wasn't messy, but the thought of having to start over made me nervous. Would I have time to find someone else, get married, and have kids before it was too late? While on the trek, I celebrated my thirty-second birthday, which wasn't necessarily old, but I wasn't a spring chicken either.

I spent time analyzing myself, specifically my past relationships and the ways in which they had or hadn't been compatible. I reflected on the things that made me happy and how important it was to have a partner who shared my interests. Throughout this process, I realized that I needed to find someone who loved the outdoors as much as I did.

I was no stranger to backpacking or mountaineering. I've been a volunteer ski patroller as part of the National Ski Patrol program for almost 20 years. For the last 7 of those, I've been the Mountain Travel and Rescue program advisor for Southern California. As part of the course, I help teach students how to survive in the backcountry, how to build and sleep in a snow cave, and how to travel safely. The time I spend volunteering for ski patrol is an important part of my life and has helped shape who I am as a person. Through ski patrol, my love of the outdoors has only grown.

What I love about being in the backcountry is that it helps you build the fortitude to get through the challenging aspects of your life. You learn how to prepare and how to problem solve. When you're having difficulty hiking, you just need to remember to put one foot in front of the other and keep going.

Here is what you learn: you realize that if you're tired, you can't just sit down and give up. You must have a strong mindset as much as physical endurance. That things taste a little sweeter when you've had to work hard to get them. The feeling of pride and joy that comes with proving you're up to the challenge is exhilarating!

A new chapter

My now husband and I met through ski patrol, and he loves the outdoors even more than I do. We've had a lot of adventures together, backpacking, rock climbing, and mountaineering, but, of course, it never seems enough. We spent our honeymoon backpacking through Patagonia, and it was unforgettable. We traveled through some of the most beautiful glaciers, mountains, lakes, and valleys in the world. Highlights included sleeping in a tent facing Mount Fitz Roy and coming face to face with a huge Guanaco (which looks like a giant llama).

Being outdoors also helps me get a sense of clarity. I am fully present with all of me. I have time to think and to process without the distractions of the phone, social media, people, and life's daily responsibilities.

Before our marriage, my husband and I were camping in the Sierras, and we were stuck in the tent during an afternoon rain shower. All we had was time: time to think and talk. It was during that conversation that I realized that I wanted to change careers. I had been in the IT field for a long time, but it dawned on me that to get the freedom I wanted, I needed to finish getting my CPA license and eventually open my own practice.

Life is like climbing: you keep climbing and climbing, and then, in an instant, you can change direction and move to the next summit, soaring even higher.

I walked away from that weekend feeling determined and with a renewed sense of purpose. A year later, I had passed all my exams and landed a job at a mid-sized accounting firm. Five years later, I branched out on my own. I would never have been able to do any of that if I hadn't stepped away from the craziness of day-to-day life and realized I needed to make a change.

Hard realizations

The Annapurna Circuit was one of the hardest and most rewarding things I had ever done. As hard as it was, it was nothing compared to the next chapter in my life.

Because of my age, my husband and I had decided to try to have children soon after our marriage. I had wanted kids my whole life and never thought that it would not happen. We found out that I was pregnant not long after.

Unfortunately, our elation didn't last long. At our seven-week appointment, we were so excited and waiting to hear our baby's heartbeat. During the ultrasound, I could see my doctor's face, and I knew something was wrong. They finally told us that they couldn't hear a heartbeat. I remember just going numb. My doctor wanted me to come back in two weeks.

I felt a bit lost. There was nothing I or my husband could do but wait until our next appointment. We had just shared the news with my parents and brother. It was a bit premature, but we were too excited to keep it to ourselves. Now, I felt like I had jinxed myself.

Our next appointment felt like a whirlwind. I had another ultrasound, and it confirmed there was no heartbeat. The next step was a D&C, a surgery to remove the fetus. We scheduled it for a few days out. I had it, then went home to recover both mentally and physically.

It was a setback, but we got through it. As soon as I was cleared medically, we tried again. We were successful a second time. My husband and I were excited but definitely a bit nervous. Once again at our seven-week appointment, we waited anxiously for the ultrasound. But it was not meant to be. I was devastated.

After two back-to-back miscarriages, we discussed options with my doctor. The results from my D&C surgeries were that my eggs were old. Old? I was only 35! The next step was to try in vitro fertilization (IVF). The thought terrified me because one of my biggest fears was blood and needles, and I knew there were lots of shots involved in IVF.

At first, I was hopeful about the process. I knew I could handle it mentally. I had done a lot of hard things (or so I thought), and I've always prided myself on being mentally tough. We really liked the IVF doctor we found, and we were going to do everything he said and it would work.

It turns out it was not so easy. In the first round we were not so successful, but we tried again, and again, and again. I began to get depressed because the realization that I might not be able to have children was slowly becoming a reality. It was hard, and it was draining, and it was difficult to pick myself up day after day and try again. But what choice did I have?

The other difficult part was that I kept it to myself. I didn't reach out to my friends for support or motivation. I relied on myself, my husband, and my parents. But outside of that circle, I stayed closed off. I had other friends getting pregnant, and I was so happy for them, but it was so hard not to be frustrated and think, "Why not me?". What had I done wrong in life that I couldn't have kids? Eventually, I decided to confide in one of my close co-workers because it was too much for me. The stress of working in a job where no one knew what was going on was difficult to manage.

IVF was a year-long, frustrating, and depressing process. But after four rounds of IVF with 292 shots, 30 blood draws, 8 surgeries, and lots of money spent, we managed to have two healthy embryos.

Looking back, I'm not sure why I kept it hidden. Maybe I didn't want people to judge, or I didn't want them to know I was struggling. It is only years later that I can openly talk about it. And I realize that it's something that should be talked about because so many people struggle with infertility. Trust me, my doctor's office was always full.

One more scare

In mountaineering, a "false summit" is a point on a mountain that appears to be the highest point, but once reached, you realize there is still a higher peak further along the trail. Essentially, a "false summit" is a deceptive peak that looks like the top but isn't.

We had two embryos, and it was time to try to implant. The first was successful! I had a fairly normal pregnancy, with some pains toward the end. When I went into labor, however, that's when things got a little scary.

It was my husband's birthday, and we were out to a celebratory dinner with friends when my contractions started. I waited until we were home to tell him because I wanted to make sure I was actually in labor. A little panicked, we both tried to get some sleep. My contractions were very irregular that night, and we went to the hospital first thing in the morning.

The nurses checked me in, ran the standard tests, and were about to send me home to wait longer. All of a sudden, their whole demeanor changed. They hooked me up to machines, tried to get an IV in me and couldn't (I was a bit dehydrated), and then spilled a box of needles on me (with my fear of needles). I didn't really know what was going on.

It turns out I had preeclampsia, and they were afraid I was going to have a stroke. That led to an emergency C-section. This was not at all what my delivery plan was supposed to be!

In the end, I was OK, and I delivered a beautiful, healthy baby boy. I had reached my true summit. Or so I thought?

It was in the months after, though, that I realized that I had lost my desire to be out in the mountains. I had no motivation to hike, work out, or plan a trip. My husband tried to get me excited, but I just got frustrated. He would come up with new workouts for me, but I would only give them half my effort. The outdoors had been such a big part of my life, and now it felt like it didn't even matter. I couldn't figure out what had happened.

The path toward healing

During Covid, my husband and I moved to Big Bear, a small mountain town outside of Los Angeles. Our son was almost one. It was then that I began to heal mentally. My journey had taken me from a year of miscarriages into a year of IVF, a year of pregnancy, motherhood, and then back to work without a breather or any time to process everything that had happened.

It was at this point that I branched out on my own and started my own accounting firm. The combination of being isolated and having a major decrease in my work allowed me to start enjoying the things I loved again. I was living in one of my favorite places, going on hikes in the forest and taking my son to play in nature. I was able to focus on myself and my family, and for that, I am eternally grateful.

Fast forward to the present day: I have two amazing children, a five-year-old boy and a three-year-old girl. They are my everything.

At three and five, our kids have been skiing, backpacking, and climbing on 100-foot rock walls. They love it, and it makes my heart smile. As they get older, we will teach them to be self-supportive by using their decision-making skills and having responsibilities when we are out on adventures. I believe that nature is a great teacher of life lessons and that these experiences will help them learn to navigate every challenge that life throws at them.

While my goal is to empower both of my children to be comfortable outside camping, backpacking, or mountaineering, I think these lessons are especially important to teach my daughter. Women underestimate themselves and their abilities in the outdoors, and I want to encourage as many women as possible to take a chance and do it. I want my daughter to know that women are tougher than people give us credit for. We can learn to be emotionally strong so that we can get through anything. We can climb any peak.

What is it that drives me?

My family and friends think I'm crazy sometimes. They sometimes roll their eyes when I say we are going camping again or that there is another climb we want to do. I think deep down, it's in my genes. My grandparents, especially my grandfather, were avid campers, rock climbers, and mountaineers in Romania.

Life continues to get more complicated. It's always difficult trying to balance raising two small children, building a career, maintaining a marriage, and keeping my sanity by playing outside.

Yet, as hard as it seems some days, I choose to let my kids wander in the forest during the day while I work at night after bedtime, and I know it's all worth it. I hope to pass on my love of the outdoors to my son and daughter and one day be able to share even bigger adventures with them.

Natalie Regg

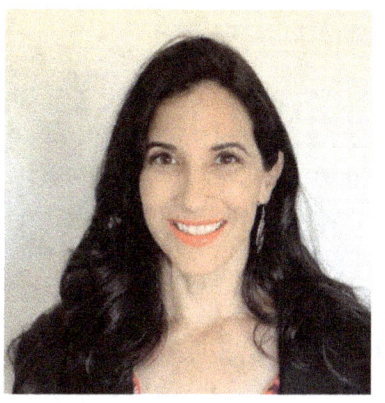

Natalie Regg is the founder of Redpoint Accounting Solutions. She is a CPA, CISA is a practicing CPA providing tax, bookkeeping, and attestation services, among other things. Natalie has been a Volunteer Ski Patroller in Big Bear for the past 17 years, providing first aid and emergency rescue. She is also a member of a Winter Search and Rescue team.

Redpoint Accounting Solutions was formed with the realization that the cannabis industry had created a need for accountants knowledgeable in cannabis tax rules. They wanted to help you navigate 280E, establish GAAP financials, and keep month-end reports accurate and current. Their goal is to find the best ways to save their clients' money.

Natalie's bookkeeping and accounting services can help maximize deductions, spend less on taxes, and offer support during audits.

Natalie Regg, CPA, CISA, is the Founder of Redpoint Accounting Solutions. Natalie enjoys helping clients grow their businesses by providing peace of mind that their finances are handled proficiently. This allows her clients to do their best: manage their business. Natalie is a Certified Public Accountant in the state of California.

When not in the office, Natalie enjoys spending time outdoors with family mountaineering, skiing, and rock climbing.

Website: http://www.redpointcpa.com/

Facebook: https://www.facebook.com/natalie.muraciov

LinkedIn: https://www.linkedin.com/in/natalie-regg-cpa

Breaking Barriers, Inspiring Change
Baydsar Thomasian

As I reflect on my extraordinary journey, I feel deeply humbled by the profound impact I have had on my long-standing career. Over two decades, I have navigated a dynamic world filled with challenges and aspiring individuals, leaving an impression on the grand City of Los Angeles and the Golden State of California.

My unwavering mission to champion dignity for all within the state deeply resonates with my tireless work to empower communities that have long yearned for recognition. Witnessing the transformative power of my zealous commitment is truly inspiring.

My name is Baydsar. Growing up in the close-knit Armenian community of Los Angeles, surrounded by a rich cultural heritage, shaped who I am today. It taught me the power of solidarity and the importance of preserving traditions. From an early age, I developed a strong fondness for family and togetherness, forming the foundation for my journey. Over the years, I faced tribulations while cherishing accomplishments and learning invaluable skills like resoluteness and persistence to guide me through life.

In my esteemed role as a political consultant to State Senator Maria Elena Durazo, I shine as a brilliant beacon of knowledge and power. I dance through the tortuous tango of politics and bureaucracy, strategically using my foresight to magnify impactful change in California's most cherished communities. My efforts have connected constituents with government initiatives that promote economic prosperity and growth while inspiring countless lives. Through spearheading benevolent projects that invigorate

Hollywood, my warmth and commitment have created lasting positive effects in the surrounding areas.

In June 2017, the Hollywood Chamber of Commerce honored me with the Hero of Hollywood Award in recognition of these efforts, a testament to my dedication to providing exceptional constituent services.

In 2019, during COVID-19, I was diagnosed and went through cancer treatment. Chemotherapy brought significant changes, including hair loss. Hats—already a personal signature—became a source of comfort and a form of self-expression. For me, they bridge the gap between vulnerability and normalcy. Since everyone knows I love wearing hats, few could differentiate whether I wore them for style or necessity. After months of treatment, I was fortunate to achieve remission. I returned with renewed strength to what fuels my passion: empowering communities and serving with purpose and determination.

My experience overcoming challenges and persevering through difficult circumstances has provided me and my family with valuable insights and empathy in my role as a political consultant. Life experiences guide us in navigating complexities and bringing people together. Just as I wore different hats during my healing journey, I approached my role as a political consultant with a similar mindset. The bottom line is that we all have the best at heart… it is what I am to wear to help facilitate and bring the like-minded together for the best results.

Remember, effective negotiation with mind and body or people with different interests often involves active listening, empathy, and understanding the motivations and priorities of each party involved. It may require finding compromises, identifying shared interests, or exploring creative solutions that meet the needs of all stakeholders.

Finding Common Ground

As an Armenian woman and a political consultant, I wear many hats—literally and metaphorically. Each role, I assume, brings unique challenges, yet they share common threads:

Adaptability: As a political consultant, you must adapt to different situations and navigate complex scenarios. Similarly, dealing with cancer requires adjusting to new challenges, treatments, and changes in your life.

Multitasking: Consultants handle various issues simultaneously, balancing interests, perspectives, and priorities. Similarly, living with cancer might involve juggling medical appointments, treatments, emotional well-being, and personal responsibilities.

Empathy and Communication: Effective negotiation requires understanding the needs and concerns of all parties involved. Empathy and clear communication are crucial in building relationships and finding common ground. Likewise, while coping with cancer, empathy towards yourself and effective communication with your healthcare team, family, and friends play a vital role.

Resilience and Determination: Negotiations can be challenging and require persistence and resilience to reach favorable outcomes. Similarly, facing cancer demands resilience, determination, and a fighting spirit to overcome physical, emotional, and psychological obstacles.

Problem-Solving: Consultants are skilled, analytical people who find creative solutions to complex issues. Likewise, dealing with cancer requires discovering solutions to medical, emotional, and practical problems that arise during the journey.

Balancing Roles: Consultants often represent different interests and work to find compromises that benefit multiple parties. Similarly, you may wear various hats, fulfilling roles as a patient, advocate, family member, or friend while finding ways to balance them all.

Continuous Learning: Political consultants constantly learn about current issues, strategies, and techniques to improve their skills. Similarly, living with cancer involves ongoing learning about your condition, treatment options, self-care, and ways to enhance your well-being.

While being a political consultant and battling cancer are distinct experiences, they share common attributes: resilience, adaptability, empathy, and problem-solving. Recognizing these similarities has allowed me to draw strength from my expertise and experiences, applying those skills to navigate both challenges successfully.

One of my shining moments was the trailblazing establishment of the LACER After School Program—a bastion of opportunity for Hollywood students. This iconic initiative provides much-needed safe and nurturing spaces for young people to learn, grow, and discover their passions. Not only do they receive robust academic support, but they also engage in exciting activities that allow them to explore their talents. Shining brightly as a beacon of hope, LACER offers students an invaluable opportunity to unlock their potential and pursue even bigger dreams.

Journey to Politics

I am committed to further empowering youth, so I actively engage with them, offering mentoring and coaching to help them succeed. Drawing from my struggles and victories, I serve as a living example, inspiring these young minds to believe that their energy and ambition can spark transformation. Faith in youth is essential for building a brighter future—an ideal I hold close to my heart.

My journey in public service began as a Field Deputy for former Councilmember Jackie Goldberg, where I worked to create something remarkable. I led the effort to establish Little Armenia, providing a cultural haven for the Armenian community, and supported the Thai community in forming Thai Town, fostering pride and unity.

Among the milestones of my career was leading a delegation to Armenia to establish a Sister City relationship between Yerevan and Los Angeles. This collaboration opened doors to cultural and economic exchange and earned me a National Honor from the Prime Minister of Armenia in September 2017 for my services to the homeland.

My work in Hollywood has also left an indelible mark. I facilitated the permitting process for the Kodak Theatre, helped transition Hollywood and Highland to host The Jimmy Kimmel Show, and secured a star on the Hollywood Walk of Fame for Charles Aznavour. In October 2017, the Charles Aznavour Foundation recognized this achievement with the Gratitude Award.

These efforts created opportunities and growth. I also brought grants to youth organizations like the Hollywood LACER After School Program, supporting their success and expansion. Through my interactions with the business community, I understood the immense power of collaboration in fostering economic growth.

Recognized as a Woman of Distinction and a Hero of Hollywood, I am committed to fostering a thriving business environment. As a political consultant for Senator Maria Elena Durazo, I advocate for influential bills, such as the Hollywood Film Tax Credits, which amplify meaningful change in communities.

My commitment extends beyond professional achievements. I collaborated on establishing the LACER After School Program, creating a safe space for Hollywood students to learn, grow, and thrive. I also served on the Armenian National Committee and Homenetmen Youth Organization boards, supporting the Armenian community and fostering cultural pride. Mentoring students at the Jesse M. Unruh Institute of Politics has become a personal mission, as I recognize their potential to create positive change.

As a District Consultant for State Senator Maria Elena Durazo, I navigate state and city bureaucracies to aid business owners and individuals in overcoming obstacles. I connect them with resources and foster partnerships that cultivate an environment where dreams can flourish. My mission is to inspire you to become part of democracy and make your voice heard for change on matters you care about.

With my deep public service and community advocacy knowledge, I know my way around politics. My journey in public service is marked by significant accomplishments, from establishing cultural havens to reshaping the landscape of Hollywood. Yet, my vision for the future transcends my success. I dream of a world where everyone can coexist peacefully, regardless of background or culture. Through my story of resilience, unwavering hope, and perseverance, I aim to encourage others to believe in themselves and join me in building a more inclusive, harmonious society where everybody is heard, valued, and empowered—so that each person's dreams can become a reality.

As I share my narrative of resilience and its impact on the world around me, I generously offer pearls of wisdom, hoping they inspire you to forge your path. I passionately advocate for believing in yourself and honoring your unique gifts, skills, and aspirations.

Celebrate every achievement with enthusiasm and recognize each step forward as a victory!

Life challenges you at every turn, but you hold a vast pool of courage and strength ready to help you overcome adversity. With an unwavering spirit, you can face the most challenging obstacles head-on and emerge transformed. Empowerment through determination—now that's something utterly worth striving for.

I share sage advice for navigating bureaucracy and creating a meaningful impact, starting in your neighborhood. You achieve powerful results by building strong relationships, uniting forces, and engaging with businesses. It's crucial to remain authentic. Listen to your heart, follow your dreams, and hold onto your beliefs. Authenticity is your most excellent power!

Throughout my journey, I have faced countless hardships that have tested my inner fortitude. During these challenging trails, I have drawn strength from the unwavering pillars of love, faith, and tradition. These foundational elements hold incredible power, enabling me to overcome even the most daunting obstacles. With heartfelt sincerity, I encourage you to tap into your spiritual essence—for within it lies the courage and inspiration to embrace your authentic self and create a lasting impact on our world.

Embracing the unknown is a transformative act that I ardently advocate. Unforeseen changes serve as remarkable opportunities for growth and self-discovery. My journey is a testament to this truth: adapting to life's unexpected twists can lead you down unexplored paths, often revealing profound personal transformation and unforeseen opportunities. So, as you navigate periods of uncertainty, approach them with an open mind — you may uncover strengths and possibilities you never imagined.

I have been fortunate to be guided by remarkable individuals and mentors who have profoundly influenced my journey. Their unwavering support, direction, and inspiration enabled me to rise above challenges and make a meaningful impact on the lives of others. I wouldn't be where I am today without them—they are the wind beneath my wings.

Bathed in the faith of my community, I strive to demonstrate how collective action can spark deep and lasting change. I remind us that all those driven souls can come together to build something monumental regardless of their backgrounds. When we unite with a shared purpose, we can effect transformative change. It begins with each of us discovering the passion that fuels our fire—whether through personal connections, organized efforts, or the inspiring resilience of those who thrive despite adversity.

With a strong focus on the future, I am fully committed to leaving behind a legacy of motivation and progress. My drive is to build a society where we can embrace our true selves, dismantle the barriers that hinder our aspirations, and nurture more cohesive communities through cooperation. It's the vision I wholeheartedly support.

In 2008, I faced health challenges that prompted me to reevaluate my career with the city. During this pivotal time, I joined forces with Councilman Eric Garcetti, embarking on a new professional journey that led me to align with Senator Kevin de León—a dedicated advocate for Hollywood's interests.

Over the following decade, I devoted myself to advancing communities by helping them navigate the complexities of government bureaucracy and resolving business-related concerns. My primary objective was to facilitate the growth of flourishing enterprises. When Kevin de León assumed the position of President pro Tempore of the California State Senate—governing one of the world's largest economies—my influence extended beyond regional boundaries and into international platforms.

In 2014, I was pivotal in persuading Kevin de León to proactively endorse California's recognition of Artsakh's independence—a region unfamiliar to many, including de León himself. This bold initiative provoked strong rebukes from the State Department and the Turkish and Azeri governments, which employed on-site visits and intimidation tactics. Despite these challenges, I remained steadfast in advocating for justice and standing by my beliefs.

In 2015, during de León's tenure as Senate President, he held the authority to nominate individuals to California State Commissions. Recognizing this invaluable opportunity, I successfully leveraged my influence to secure appointments for six Armenians in these roles. This achievement echoed the era of Governor George Deukmejian when the Armenian community held noteworthy influence. It inspired immense pride within the community and underscored the enduring impact of dedicated advocacy.

Bridging the Gap

In politics, deputy positions are inherently transient, tied to the tenure of elected officials. These roles lack union protections and often face precarious circumstances. Despite these challenges, I have survived and thrived within the Hollywood District, dedicating 29 years to this demanding arena. Throughout this journey, I have worked under the leadership of influential figures, including Councilman Mike Woo, Councilmember Jackie Goldberg, Senator Kevin de León, and now Senator Maria Elena Durazo. Each leader representing Hollywood since 1994 has significantly shaped my experiences and growth in public service.

Each role has been an opportunity to advocate for meaningful change, build relationships, and contribute to the community's progress while overcoming the challenges accompanying such dynamic positions.

Working on an international scale has allowed me to address significant issues and make a lasting impact on California politics. Reflecting on these experiences fills me with immense gratitude for my opportunities to empower communities and advocate for positive change. As we conclude my story's conclusion, a profound sense of accomplishment and appreciation emerges. I have crafted every chapter of this journey to leave an enduring impression not only on myself but, I hope, on others as well. Yet, this tale is more than just a reflection of one person's achievements. It invites you to embrace your own path—with zest, ambition, and unwavering dedication to making a difference.

I encourage you to celebrate the journey that is your life. Reflect on moments of joy, the successes you've achieved, and the challenges you've overcome. Remember those who have walked alongside you at various times. Every step forward, every kind act for others, and every leap of growth is part of a greater celebration—one we should all take pride in!

In this grand finale, let us remember that each one of us can make an invaluable contribution to our shared humanity. Never underestimate the profound and lasting impact we can have on the lives of others and our own. With faith in ourselves and confidence in our unique voices and perspectives, we create ripples of change —lifting spirits, inspiring others, and transforming communities for the better.

Despite coping with health issues, the remarkable journey of women rising to higher positions is a testament to their resilience and unwavering determination. You, too, can be one of the trailblazers, navigating life's complexities with grace and grit.

As the curtain falls on my story, I hope it leaves your heart stirred by what we can achieve through bravery, strength, and kindness. Let my message resonate:

- Cherish your journey.
- Honor your victories.
- Embrace the limitless possibilities within yourself—because the world needs your unique voice.
- Appreciate every single person.
- Ensure everyone has an equal opportunity to reach their goals.

Together, let us strive to create a brighter, more inclusive future.

Baydsar Thomasian!

Baydsar Thomasian

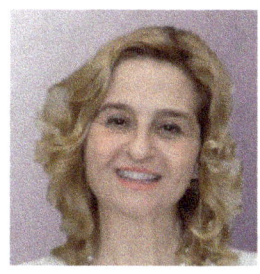

Baydsar Thomasian is the Political Consultant to California Senator Maria Elena Durazo. Her career spans over two decades of impactful public service to Hollywood, the City of Los Angeles, and the State of California. She has served as Hollywood Field Deputy for former Councilmember Jackie Goldberg, Senior Field Deputy for former Council President Eric Garcetti, and Deputy District Director for Senate President Pro Tem Kevin De Leon. She is currently a Political Consultant to Senator Maria Elena Durazo.

Baydsar's work as a veteran public servant has left an indelible mark on every organization in the Hollywood and Armenian communities. Born in Armenia and raised in Los Angeles, she is the first Armenian immigrant deputy who has served the City of Hollywood area for over two decades. Her inspiring leadership in 1999 led to the creation of Little Armenia and helped the Thai Community create Thai Town. This City Designation sparked years of Armenian Genocide marches, commemoration events, and festivals.

Throughout her career, Baydsar has been a beacon of hope and encouragement, mentoring minorities, immigrants, disadvantaged youth, and other segments of our community on empowerment and engagement. Beyond her professional commitments, Baydsar is a dedicated mother and wife who volunteers at non-profit organizations in her community and mentors young adults seeking to improve their academic skills. She has also served on the Board of the prestigious Jesse M. Unruh Institute of Politics at USC as an Ambassador, guiding students to make a difference in society. In 2006, Johnny Grant nominated her for the Women of Distinction Award.

Instagram: https://www.instagram.com/baydsarthomasian/

LinkedIn: https://www.linkedin.com/in/baydsar-thomasian-8b496915

Guided by Faith
A JOURNEY OF RESILIENCE, COMPASSION, AND INSPIRATION
Irma Villegas

My name is Irma Villegas, and my story begins in the serene landscapes of Jalisco, Mexico, on a small farm named El Colomo. It was a place where time seemed to slow down, and traditions were passed down through generations. My parents, Maria and Alberto, were no exception to this enduring legacy. Both were born in El Colomo, and our family had been cattle farmers as far back as anyone could remember. But destiny had other plans for my father.

Alberto was a young man with aspirations beyond the simplicity of farm life. He yearned for a better future that the United States promised with its allure of opportunities and possibilities. So, with hope in his heart, he left Mexico, embarking on a journey to the land of dreams. In the United States, my father worked hard, toiling in various jobs to make a life for himself. He would travel back and forth to visit our family in Mexico, keeping the connection between the two worlds alive. On one of these visits, he met my mother, Maria, and their love story began to unfold. They got married and started a family together.

New Beginnings

When I was born, my mother had a heart-to-heart conversation with my father, urging him to take us to the United States. She knew that life in Mexico, although deeply rooted in tradition, would offer limited opportunities for her children. With a great sense of responsibility, my father agreed, and we began our journey to the United States.

Our visa secured our passage, and we crossed the border in Nogales, Arizona. Initially excited to start a new life, we hardly realized that our visa would expire soon after my brother's birth. Nevertheless, we pressed forward, facing the challenges that lay ahead.

As a young girl in a foreign land, I struggled to adapt to my new surroundings. The language barrier was one of the most daunting obstacles, and I needed help to speak English fluently. The other kids at school teased me for my Mexican heritage, making me feel like an outsider in my community.

Amidst the difficulties, I found solace in a friendship that blossomed during recess and after school. My newfound friend, who also spoke Spanish, became my guide, patiently teaching me English and helping me navigate cultural differences. With his support, I started to find my place in this new world, bridging the gap between my old and new identities.

Every summer, my family and I traveled back to Mexico to visit my Abuelita on my mother's side. She was a devoted Catholic, and her life revolved around her faith. Abuelita prayed daily, and I remember her carrying a small school picture of me in her apron, saying she prayed for me all day. As a child, I couldn't fully comprehend the depth of her devotion, but I knew in my heart that her prayers were guiding me in some mysterious way. By this time, we had acquired our Green Card as a family. I later became a US Citizen.

Time passed, and our family moved to Glendale when I was twelve years old. My father worked diligently to find employment, while my mother joined him in supporting the family. Life was far from easy, but they did their best with what they had to provide for us.

As I entered 11th grade, my parents' marriage began to crumble under the weight of my father's battle with alcoholism. The emotional toll on our family was immense, and the burden of financial responsibility fell on my sister and me. We lived in a modest two-bedroom apartment and had to grow up quickly to shoulder the responsibilities of supporting our three younger siblings.

During those tumultuous times, I found solace in walking the football field at school during zero-period PE. There, I encountered a kind-hearted man, a stranger who would unknowingly change the course of my life. We started a conversation, and I poured out my heart, sharing the raw emotions surrounding my family's struggles. To my surprise, he revealed he was a Family Therapist and listened to me with empathy and understanding. He would then say something I have kept until now, "You are the sanest person I know." He assured me that my feelings were valid and that many families face similar challenges. His comforting words resonated deep within me, and I felt a strange sense of peace—a peace that I later attributed to the prayers of my Abuelita. This encounter shifted my perspective on my life.

Soon after high school, I pursued my passion for food and took a different path than the traditional route of attending college. I began an apprenticeship with a pastry chef, immersing myself in pastry-making for two years. I fell in love with culinary arts, and my passion for the food business flourished. That passion led me to open a small coffee and sandwich restaurant in the heart of Hollywood. The restaurant was a dream come true, but financial difficulties and differences with my partner eventually led to its closure. Although it may have seemed like a failure, I took it as a valuable learning experience, gaining insights into finance and business operations. From sourcing vendors and remodeling the space to finding equipment and working long hours, that first entrepreneurial venture taught me invaluable lessons.

After the restaurant's closure, I transitioned to working with a Five-Star chef in a professional kitchen. The opportunity to cook for celebrities was thrilling, but I soon realized that the job felt lonely and disconnected. Spending long hours in the kitchen prepping for the night and not getting the chance to interact with clients during service left me unfulfilled. I took a deep breath and realized I loved people more than the food itself. This realization prompted me to make a change, and I soon began working as a manager at a restaurant at UCLA. Running a restaurant spanning over 20,000 square feet for the students was challenging and rewarding. I knew this was where life would change. And yes, I met my future husband, Carlos. He had recently graduated from UCLA and was also a Restaurant Student Manager at a different restaurant. Our paths crossed, and we started dating and married four years later.

With Carlos by my side, we created a 10-year timeline, carefully planning our finances and career goals. We sought guidance from mentors and educators who played instrumental roles in educating us on financial matters. Thanks to their support, we learned how to eliminate consumer debt, school loans, and car loans while purchasing homes.

Carlos secured a job with the City of Los Angeles, and with the stability of our careers, we could plan for our family. Our two daughters, Mia and Ella, are beautiful young girls and our most outstanding teachers.

Motherhood has brought me immense joy and a renewed determination to secure our family's stable and prosperous future. I became obsessed with learning how to make more money and plan for our future, taking numerous finance classes to expand my knowledge. My thirst for understanding led me to H&R Block, where I enrolled in a tax preparation course and became a certified tax preparer. Working three seasons in the tax industry provided insights into our finances and allowed me to assist others in navigating their tax obligations.

I noticed a common thread among the wealthiest individuals – many had a Schedule E rental property. This observation piqued my interest in real estate, so I obtained my real estate license. With a new skill set, I ventured into the world of real estate.

In 2016, I began my philanthropic journey by joining Glendale Kiwanis. My time with the Glendale Kiwanis opened my eyes to the joy and fulfillment of community service. As a child, I received support from various nonprofits, such as gifts from the police station and food from the Salvation Army. As a fortunate homeowner with financial independence, I strongly desire to give back to my community.

One of my most impactful volunteering experiences was with my daughters during the Cop for Kids Toy Drive organized by the Glendale Police Department in 2018. Assigned to deliver toys, food, and even a Christmas tree to needy families, I was handed a piece of paper with an address.

To my astonishment, the address was for the same little apartment where we had lived when we first arrived in Glendale. Memories of our struggles in that apartment came rushing back, but instead of feeling emotional, I was overwhelmed with gratitude. It was a profound moment of realization, connecting the dots between my past and present and reaffirming my faith in the guiding force that had brought me to this point in life.

Today, I continue to work diligently in real estate, striving for success and financial security for my family. My journey has been filled with challenges, faith, and the unwavering support of those around me. As a mother, wife, entrepreneur, and philanthropist, I am grateful for every experience that has shaped me and led me to where I am today. My faith and the prayers of my Abuelita have been my guiding lights, providing strength and direction as I navigate life's twists and turns. With determination and gratitude, I embrace all the joys and challenges that come my way, always staying true to the values instilled in me by my family and my faith.

Looking back on my life, I am filled with profound gratitude. From my humble beginnings on a farm in Jalisco to becoming an advocate for my community, my life's path has been shaped by faith. Through all the ups and downs, I held on to the belief in a guiding force, propelling me on a path of resilience, compassion, and inspiration. I can see how faith has intertwined itself with every step I've taken. The unwavering thread that held me together during the darkest times and the beacon of hope that led me toward the light. Faith was the guiding force that helped me navigate the challenges of a new country, the struggles of a broken family, and the uncertainty of my future.

Today, I dedicate myself to family and serving others. I know that no matter how challenging life may be, having faith in oneself and a higher power can light the way to an authentic and inspirational journey. My story is a testament to the power of faith, showing how it can transform lives and bring light to the darkest corners of our hearts.

I am reminded of the prayers of my Abuelita, who never stopped believing in the power of faith to shape destinies and heal hearts. I carry her legacy with me, and I know I am living proof of the miracles that can happen when guided by faith.

Looking back on my life

My experiences have taught me that faith is not just about religious beliefs but a profound trust in the universe and ourselves. It is the unwavering conviction that there is a purpose to every challenge we face, and that hope is waiting to be discovered even in the depths of despair. Faith is the anchor that keeps us grounded during life's storms and the wings that carry us to new heights when we dare to dream.

Volunteering allows me to meet people from diverse backgrounds, each with struggles and triumphs. I see families living in poverty, battling hardships much like my own family had once faced. Yet, amidst the struggles, I witness their unwavering faith in a brighter tomorrow. Their resilience and determination to overcome obstacles for a better future.

Volunteering with Glendale Kiwanis, I have the privilege of collaborating with incredible individuals dedicated to making a difference. We unite under the banner of faith, sharing a common vision of a compassionate and harmonious world.

My life has been a testament to the resilience of the human spirit and the unwavering power of faith to lead us toward our purpose.

Faith is my guiding light; I am filled with gratitude for the blessings in my life. I have a loving family, a supportive community, and a purpose-driven life that allows me to be of service to others. Each day, I am humbled by the opportunity to positively impact the lives of those around me, just as my Abuelita and the Family Therapist did for me.

To those who are facing their trials and tribulations, I offer this message of hope:

1. No matter how challenging life may seem, have faith in yourself and the universe.

2. Embrace your strength and trust that every step you take leads you towards a greater purpose.

3. Remember that even in the darkest times, a guiding force is ready to lift you and carry you toward the light.

Guided by Faith

I stand as a testament to the miraculous transformation that can occur when we wholeheartedly believe in the power of resilience, compassion, and love. As I look back on my life's journey, I know that faith has been the unwavering companion that has walked beside me every step. With faith in my heart, I continue to navigate the path ahead, knowing that no matter what lies ahead, I am guided by a force greater than myself—a force that connects us all, regardless of our backgrounds, beliefs, or circumstances.

And so, my journey of resilience, compassion, and inspiration continues, fueled by the guiding light of faith. As I move forward, I carry the legacy of my Abuelita's prayers, the wisdom of the Family Therapist's words, and the strength of all those who have walked this path before me. I stand as a testament to the power of resilience and the boundless potential within each of us.

I will continue to illuminate the world with the light of compassion and love. As my story intertwines with the stories of others, I hope that together, we can create a tapestry of hope that transcends borders and unites us in a shared vision of a brighter, more compassionate world.

Through faith, we discover the courage to rise above our challenges and the capacity to extend a hand to those in need. As my journey unfolds, faith will always guide me toward a life of purpose, compassion, and love.

Irma Villegas

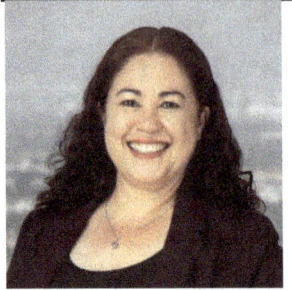

Irma Villegas is an esteemed Realtor based in Glendale, California, renowned for her three-decade-long career as a serial entrepreneur and her unwavering dedication to community service. Irma has proven herself to be a tenacious and innovative business leader with a diverse portfolio of successful ventures, including ownership of a restaurant and a multi-level marketing company.

Irma's entrepreneurial spirit is evident in her latest endeavor—a groundbreaking digital platform tailored exclusively for Spanish-speaking business owners. This platform is a testament to her passion for fostering growth and empowering entrepreneurs within her community.

Beyond her professional pursuits, Irma is deeply committed to positively impacting her community. Her involvement with esteemed organizations such as the Glendale Kiwanis Club, Glendale Latino Association, MACH Mujeres Ativas En El Commercial Hispano, and The Tony Robbins Organization exemplifies her dedication to community service and empowerment.

Embracing a personal philosophy that true fulfillment is derived from giving back, Irma has become a driving force behind numerous community-oriented initiatives. Her selfless contributions have earned her respect and admiration from her peers and community members.

Facebook: https://www.facebook.com/irma.villegas/

Instagram: https://www.instagram.com/theirmavillegas/

LinkedIn: https://www.linkedin.com/in/irma-villegas-b12a1a13/

To Armenia, with Love

Liana Tomekyan

During my first four years in Armenia, I was too young to remember how difficult it was for my parents, but just hearing the stories, seeing the photo albums, and meeting my relatives made it like I was there in person. Growing up in southern California was a long way from Armenia. The memories of the Armenian genocide and the hardships my fellow Armenians faced were etched into the faces of my parents and grandparents. Still, they refused to be defined by them. I lived through and empathized with those struggles, looking through my parents' eyes. Seeing my parents work hard, be entrepreneurial, and create opportunities not just for themselves but for many friends and family in the US and back in Armenia has made me who I am today.

My parents didn't know English, so we received government assistance to get our start. But more than that, my parents were determined to ensure we succeeded. I was in the parking lot of our apartment complex serving coffee to my dad's automotive repair customers. He always had a waiting list of customers lined up from Hollywood to Santa Monica to get in to see my dad with their cars. Mom and Dad were always wise with their time and their resources. Mom was attending school while working and caring for the home and family.

My Son, the Entrepreneur

I'm so proud of my son, who's now 16 and a Junior in High School. Inspired by his grandparents, his dad, and myself, he thinks and acts like an entrepreneur. Through the years, he's watched me build my financial services business, a hospice business, and I am currently running a nonprofit organization with a dear friend of mine, Mariam "Mary" Kavukchyan, whom we met during the war in Armenia.

It is heartwarming and encouraging to see him follow in our families' footsteps in starting, operating, and growing multiple businesses and streams of income. Some say children learn by listening, but we all learn by watching and following suit in our family. The saving grace for parents struggling with their kids right now is to continue to show by example what is right - and hope that eventually, your kids will find their path, if not follow yours.

Working in the corporate world as a single mother taught me quickly that waiting for someone else to acknowledge my work and give me a raise was not the path I wanted to take. I always wanted to work for myself, and being told "no" by a company gave me the exact courage to quit my job and start my own business! Working for myself is one of the best things I did.

Everyone has a story to share, and it's not just the story that is so compelling, but it's what each one has faced through insurmountable odds.

Diagnosed with Cancer

Being diagnosed with cancer is not something I was not prepared for, especially not in my twenties. Sitting in the doctor's office and hearing the news shocked my entire being... it was then that struck me... "I may die."

My parents, family, and my husband then gave me much inspiration.

Because of what I had to face and my positive attitude, I found more meaning and purpose in my work. I attribute my recovery to all the positive energy and vibe from friends and family who supported me during these trying times. You think you are not prepared to face a challenge like this, but the reality is that you are more resilient than you realize. And family and those who love you will help you find your inner resolve and peace to weather the storm. In fact, during this time, I chose not to read any articles about cancer and chemotherapy. Instead, I only focused on positive thoughts, my work, healing, and my future.

My Strength from Family

During my treatment, I found yet another passion – cooking. I'd have family and friends over, and no matter how frail I was, I would go to the kitchen, cook, and serve them. Connecting with friends and family like this gave me the power and the will to live and carry on. On day four of the chemo treatment, I invited some close family and friends over for some much-needed soul talk. What they did not know is how much their attentiveness and care helped strengthen and give me the will to not only kick cancer but also reboot my career and entire life. What I had been doing was writing!

My First Book 'SPRINGFIELD' was born out of this and is set in Armenia.

Cancer is a challenging and often life-altering experience, both physically and emotionally. Engaging in activities that brought me joy and purpose contributed to my overall well-being during and after the treatments. Although I would have some difficult days, cooking provided comfort, creativity, and nourishment. Exploring new recipes, experimenting with flavors, and sharing meals with loved ones can be therapeutic and uplifting.

My First Book, SPRINGFIELD, is Set in Armenia

A Little Course in Dreams, published by Beyond Publishing, follows the journey of courageous women who find a way to use their resources to help others put their lives together after suffering abuse at the hands of others. Springfield is not just a place; it is an attitude that changes the relationships and futures of all it touches. Please find out how women of means bond together to help those in need and, through the process, learn about themselves.

My Nonprofit in Armenia

I titled this chapter Back to Armenia with Love because our nonprofit Satik's Home is named after my aunt, Mary, who lost her way too early. Satik inspired her so much that we wanted to name our nonprofit after her. Satik's home, our nonprofit, is home-based in Armenia. The construction is due to start by the end of this year. (Satik, a woman's name in Armenian)

Supporting women who have lost their husbands during the war is a compassionate and meaningful endeavor. These women often face unique challenges as they navigate grief, loss, and the rebuilding of their lives. Offering them support and assistance can make a significant difference.

Our nonprofit will help young women who become widowed because of the recent Armenian war with therapy, housing, and support to complete their education and provide Armenian textiles and products so they can produce fashionable pieces to sell in Armenia and the United States. This will help generate income and revenue for the nonprofit and women who come to Satik's Home.

You could also consider volunteering with organizations that focus on helping war widows or connecting with local support groups to offer your skills and provide emotional support.

Speaking About Resilience

The resilience of these women we work with in Armenia has inspired me to do more. They are so strong and courageous even though they have lost their husbands in the war. They are determined to create a better life for themselves and their children. They've inspired me to become an advocate and speak about Satik's Home everywhere I go. I've been speaking on stage at conferences and events all over the USA, virtually online and in person. I've talked to small and large groups, corporate sponsors, and individuals who want to help make a difference. People can follow my Instagram to learn more and directly message me to learn how to donate to Satik's Home at Instagram.com/LianaTomekyan. You can contact me on Instagram to speak on your podcast, radio show, or stage about women's empowerment, overcoming adversity, or successful startups.

Honoring My Dad

I lost my dad on April 28th of this year. Believe it or not, this was far harder on me than beating cancer. I adored him. One of the most important things he instilled in me was never quitting. He gave me the greatest compliment before he passed when he held my hand and said, "You are just like me." My dad worked up to the day he died. He found so much joy and purpose in his work, which is the best way to live. He added value to the people he met by over-delivering what he promised. He instilled the same integrity and spirit of excellence in me. I believe I am who I am today because of him. I miss you, Dad, and I love you always!

Liana Tomekyan

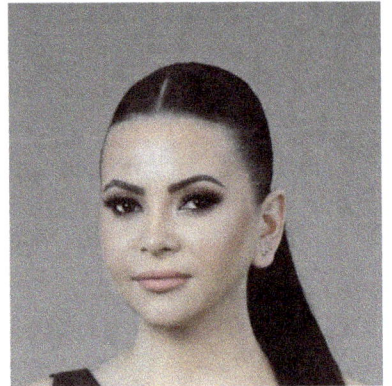

Liana Tomekyan started her journey in financial services in 2016. Fast forward to 2020. She now has many working with her in her organization.

In only a year, Liana proved to herself and others that she could lead a successful business and balance motherhood. Even as a single mother, she could lead multiple enterprises while prioritizing her son.

Liana Tomekyan started her journey in financial services in 2016. Fast forward to 2020. She now has her organization.

In only a year, Liana proved to herself and others that she could lead a successful business and balance motherhood. Even as a single mother, she led multiple enterprises while prioritizing her son.

Liana was a cancer survivor in her 20s and a single parent in her 30s after her divorce. Going through those hardships and scares is the primary reason she wants women today to know that life doesn't stop because of bumps in the road. The times when you find yourself alone, remind yourself and give yourself the strength to become who you are meant to be.

Liana Tomekyan wants to help people achieve their financial goals, just as she did for herself so that she can leave a legacy for her son. Her love for helping people and her community makes her passionate about what she does.

In addition to financial services, Liana is also a co-author of the best-selling book *Powerful Female Immigrants*.

Facebook: https://www.facebook.com/lianatomekyanfinancialservices/
Instagram: https://www.instagram.com/lianatomekyan/
LinkedIn: https://www.linkedin.com/in/liana-t-b259a611a

"Healing may not be so much about getting better as about letting go of everything that isn't you - all of the expectations, all of the beliefs - and becoming who you are." - Rachel Naomi Remen.

About the Author

Liza Boubari is a transformational speaker, clinical hypnotherapist, and founder of HealWithin. With over 25 years of experience, she has empowered countless individuals to heal emotionally and physically, embrace their authentic selves, and evolve into the lives they truly desire. Liza's mission is to help women connect deeply with their inner strength, break free from limitations, and rediscover their worth and voice.

To learn more or connect with Liza, email her at liza.boubari@thepowerfulshe.com.

Discover More from Liza Boubari

Explore Liza's other books and recordings:

- *Stand Up to Slim Down*: Discover the link between emotional weight and physical wellness.

- *HealThy Mind-Body*: Heal within through imagination, intention, and guided imagery.

- *Stomp on Smoking*: Free yourself from smoking and emotional cravings.

- 12 self-hypnosis audio recordings available at **healwithin.com/shop**.

Tune in to *Real-talk with Liza* on AM870 at via your favorite podcast directory, including Spotify, iHeart, or on your smart Amazon device. *Real-Talk with Liza*, where candid conversations meet real experts and genuine insights.

www.ingramcontent.com/pod-product-compliance
Lightning Source LLC
Chambersburg PA
CBHW052140070526
44585CB00017B/1915